Clinical Small Animal Care

Promoting Patient Health through Preventative Nursing

Companion website

This book is accompanied by a companion website:

www.wiley.com/go/wuestenberg

The website includes:
- Powerpoints of all figures from the book for downloading
- Editable Word files containing the general forms found in Appendix 4
- Powerpoint files containing the employee skill and knowledge advancement plans found in Appendix 5

Clinical Small Animal Care

Promoting Patient Health through Preventative Nursing

Kimm Wuestenberg, CVT, VTS (ECC, SAIM)

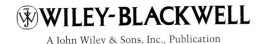

A John Wiley & Sons, Inc., Publication

This edition first published 2012 © 2012 by John Wiley & Sons, Inc.

Wiley-Blackwell is an imprint of John Wiley & Sons, formed by the merger of Wiley's global Scientific, Technical and Medical business with Blackwell Publishing.

Registered office: John Wiley & Sons Ltd, The Atrium, Southern Gate, Chichester, West Sussex, PO19 8SQ, UK

Editorial offices: 2121 State Avenue, Ames, Iowa 50014-8300, USA
The Atrium, Southern Gate, Chichester, West Sussex, PO19 8SQ, UK
9600 Garsington Road, Oxford, OX4 2DQ, UK

For details of our global editorial offices, for customer services and for information about how to apply for permission to reuse the copyright material in this book please see our website at www.wiley.com/wiley-blackwell.

Library of Congress Cataloging-in-Publication Data
Wuestenberg, Kimm.
    Clinical small animal care : promoting patient health through preventative nursing / Kimm Wuestenberg.
        p. ; cm.
    Includes bibliographical references and index.
    ISBN 978-0-8138-0514-6 (pbk. : alk. paper)
    I. Title.
    [DNLM: 1. Animal Diseases-nursing.   2. Patient Care-veterinary.   3. Veterinary Medicine-methods.   SF 774.5]
    636.089'073-dc23
                        2011037206

A catalogue record for this book is available from the British Library.

Wiley also publishes its books in a variety of electronic formats. Some content that appears in print may not be available in electronic books.

Set in 9/12.5 pt Interstate Light by Toppan Best-set Premedia Limited
Printed and bound in Malaysia by Vivar Printing Sdn Bhd

Disclaimer

1 2012

Contents

Companion website

This book is accompanied by a companion website:

www.wiley.com/go/wuestenberg

The website includes:
- Powerpoints of all figures from the book for downloading
- Editable Word files containing the general forms found in Appendix 4
- Powerpoint files containing the employee skill and knowledge advancement plans found in Appendix 5

Preface

I will always remember my very first patient suffering from multiple organ dysfunction syndrome (MODS), Angel. Looking back, I'm sure I had actually observed MODS dozens of times before Angel, but I remember her because I learned an invaluable lesson from her that night. In that 13-hour shift, I was given the opportunity to take patient care to the next level. As I cared for her, I also learned what her body was doing physically, from the sequence of dysfunctional microvascular blood flow to internal organ deterioration. I learned the common pathway of the disease process and more importantly, what measures we could take in attempts to stop the process. That night I learned that critical thinking skills, anticipation of ensuing body processes, and hands-on nursing were the true skill and talent of a veterinary technician.

Patient care and husbandry is one of the noblest nursing tasks that we have; however, it is often underrated or overlooked. Veterinary support staff members have numerous resources to use in educating themselves on particular body systems and diseases, diagnostics, therapeutics, and even performing procedures. Unfortunately, there are few resources that focus on the crucial standards of hands-on patient care. The veterinary profession as a whole has not developed a set standard of care as the human nursing field has; knowledge in this area is typically gained through experience, at the troubled expense of the patient. I recall seeing red rings of bacteria in food and water dishes when I was new to the field in 1993. I remember midcareer the patients who had lost toes and limbs due to improper bandaging techniques. More recently, in 2009, I saw a patient with an intravenous catheter site abscess and another patient with excrement scald. In essence, this equates to nearly two decades of observing a challenging enigma in this profession—the inability for veterinary practices and personnel to uphold fundamental hygiene, patient care, and nursing standards. A clean pet is a happy pet. A veterinary patient receiving proper nursing care has a better chance at recovery because of those nursing interventions.

In my own personal experiences, I have learned that turning away from a patient receiving a blood transfusion is not a good idea. I have learned that a medication dose you've asked for may not necessarily be the dose you're actually giving, so it is best to use the check system. I have underestimated the temperature of a heat source; conversely, I have underestimated the physiological effects of hypothermia. I have learned, and I will continue to learn. We all must continue to build our talents, recognize the powerful skill in our thinking and with ambition, dedication, and a true love for animals, and with this profession, be the best that we can possibly be for these precious patients we are fortunate enough to care for.

I would like to thank you, the reader, for your contribution to this profession, your devotion, and your passion for veterinary nursing.

Kimm Wuestenberg

Acknowledgments

First and foremost, I would like to thank the person who introduced me to veterinary medicine, Pam Gardner. My wonderful instructor who was faced with the challenge of teaching veterinary nursing to a 17-year-old high school student in 1993 and not only succeeded, but became one of the most influential people in my career.

I would like to thank Margaret Mills for taking me under her wing and setting the stage for future accomplishments; Jim Minnick for not only teaching me how to perform a thoracocentesis 6 months out of school, but for telling me that I *should* be performing advanced procedures as a technician; Raegan Wells, Rich Fisher, and Bill Gooldy for setting an example of how to be an all-around better person and professional; Amy Felock for sharing my passion for veterinary nursing, encouraging me, supporting me, and being the best friend a girl could have; Linda Merrill, you are an absolute inspiration and I'm honored to know you. Thanks to the Academy of Veterinary Emergency & Critical Care Technicians (AVECCT) and the Academy of Internal Medicine for Veterinary Technicians (AIMVT) for bringing so much to my life, my career, and this fantastic profession.

Lastly, I would like to thank my family whom I love dearly with all my heart: my beloved father, Richard, whose words to me throughout his life were "You can do anything, Kimberly!" and so I did; my supportive mother, Gale, who recognized my full potential before I did; my brother, Jason, for the sibling rivalry that encouraged me to always go one step further; my sister-in-law, Melissa, whose compassion and love for animals has inspired me. Most of all, I would like to thank my beautiful sons, Imre Albrecht and Kayden Avery, for all the joy, love, laughter, challenges, adventures, and growth you bring to my life . . . you are both so very special, I love you and I thank you for enriching my life.

K.W.

Clinical Small Animal Care

Promoting Patient Health
through Preventative Nursing

Clinical Fundamentals in Promoting Good Health

Chapter 1
The Elements of Environmental Husbandry

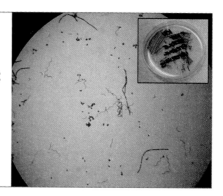

Nursing care of the veterinary patient involves astute knowledge of normal anatomy and physiology, a clear understanding of disease pathology, and practical critical thinking skills. However, a key nursing aspect often overlooked is basic nursing care of the patient and the patients' environment. Influences such as noise, temperature, hygiene, and surface area cleaning protocols can influence the heath of the patient. For example, a postoperative patient experiencing hypothermia is at risk for delayed healing, pain, surgical site infection, and a longer hospital stay, which means a possibility of developing a nosocomial infection. This section will cover basic nursing skills which have a profound affect on the patients' ability to recover from illness.

Nosocomial infections

Nosocomial infections are those that occur within the hospital setting, often referred to as "hospital-acquired" infections. They are also known as "super infections" or "super bugs," since nosocomial infections pose a great threat to the debilitated and immunocompromised veterinary patient. Microorganisms such as bacteria take Darwin's "survival of the fittest" theory to the next level when it comes to multiple antibiotic resistances in a hospital setting. They not only survive, they thrive, and veterinary patients can fatally fall victim to these "super bugs." Human medicine hospital rates for nosocomial infections tend to be higher in intensive or critical care settings; however, incidence is not limited to these areas. In addition, human nosocomial infections tend to be one of the leading causes of death in the intensive care unit (ICU) due to causing septic shock and subsequent multiple organ failure. Surprisingly, sources of nosocomial infections are the patient and the healthcare worker.

Pathogens such as *Escherichia coli*, *Pseudamonas* spp., *Acinetobacter* spp., *Serratia* spp., *Enterobacter* spp., and *Klebsiella* spp. are common culprits of nosocomial infections. More recently, methicillin-resistant *Staphylococcus aureus* (MRSA), methicillin-resistant *Staphylococcus intermedius* (MRSI), vancomycin-resistant *Staphylococcus*

Clinical Small Animal Care: Promoting Patient Health through Preventative Nursing, First Edition. Kimm Wuestenberg.
© 2012 John Wiley & Sons, Inc. Published 2012 by John Wiley & Sons, Inc.

aureus (VRSA), and vancomycin-resistant *Enterococci* (VRE) have made way to veterinary practices. Sources for these infections include (but are not limited to) venous access sites, urinary catheter sites, and surgical sites or wounds. Maintenance and handling of access sites is an essential part of veterinary patient nursing when it comes to prevention of nosocomial infection and is discussed in the section "Proper Care of Tubes and Catheters."

Preventing nosocomial infection is a simple task; however, compliance tends to be the challenge. The single most effective way to prevent a nosocomial infection is hand washing. Veterinary personnel who do not wash hands between patients virtually become fomites and transfer microorganisms from one patient to another. When these microorganisms are transferred to an ill or injured patient, the effects can be devastating due to the compromised immune system of the patient. Hand washing mechanically removes debris and transient microorganisms. A non-antimicrobial soap should be used, as resistance to an antimicrobial soap can build. Warm water should be used during a thorough wash and the hands dried completely, either with paper towels or a hot air dryer.

In addition to hand washing, the patients' housing should be properly disinfected at least every 24 hours, more frequently as needed (soiling with urine, feces, vomit, blood, etc.). The patients' bedding should also follow these guidelines, being changed or washed at least every 24 hours. Soiled bedding should be removed immediately and replaced with fresh, clean bedding. A visual surveillance of the patients' immediate environment should be frequent, ensuring a clean housing area at all times.

A microbiological surveillance plan should be established for every practice. Disinfectants and detergents can be placed on a rotating schedule to prevent resistance from developing. In addition, samples for laboratory culture can be taken from surfaces such as exam tables, surgical tables, kennels, and kennel doors as well as containers holding products used on patients (cleansers, gauze, etc.) to monitor the hospital environment for potential pathogens (Fig. 1.1).

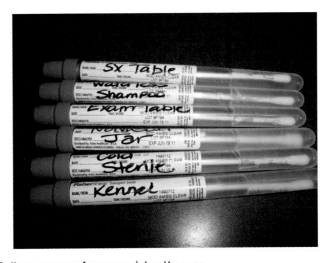

Figure 1.1 Culture survey of nosocomial pathogens.

Bedding and dish rotation

General standards for kennel cleaning include providing fresh bedding and complete disinfecting of the kennel at least once in a 24-hour period, more frequently if needed. Everything should be removed from the kennel prior to cleaning, including wastes. Kennels should be cleaned first from the top, then the sides, and finally the bottom. The kennel doors should be cleaned inside and out. Large runs should be power washed and a squeegee used to remove excess water. It is recommended to deep clean all kennels and cages once a week and rotate disinfectants to prevent nosocomial infections.

Bedding materials may range from mats, paper, sheets, towels, or blankets. Patients requiring long-term care or those with a decreased ability to ambulate should have thick bedding to prevent decubital ulcers. Although blankets and towels provide warmth and comfort to the patient, it is essential for the nursing staff to maintain cleanliness of these materials. They should be checked, both visually and by touch, to ensure the material has not been soiled. Soiled materials should be removed from the kennel, the kennel disinfected, and fresh bedding material placed. Providing comfortable, clean bedding to the patient may require more work; however, the benefits to the patient are dynamic (Fig. 1.2).

Cats and smaller dogs may feel more comfortable when given a bed to rest in. A towel can be rolled up and placed in a circular shape. Adding a small box to a kennel may also reduce stress for some cats as some prefer to remain hidden (Fig. 1.3).

Dishes should be rotated at least every 24 hours or more frequently if needed. Dried food material or contaminated water remaining in dishes may contribute to bacteria growth and illness. Once food remains at room temperature for 2 hours, it begins to grow bacteria in rapid numbers. Food left out may begin to have a strong odor or may change in consistency (sticky, slimy, etc.), indicating bacteria growth. It is best to discard food not consumed within 2 hours and store perishable diets in a refrigerator at 40°F. Bacteria may still grow in this temperature so all food should be inspected prior to feeding.

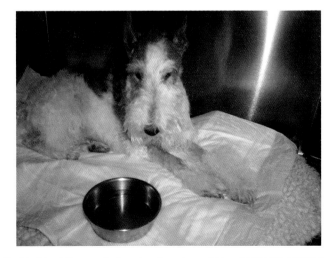

Figure 1.2 Padded bedding and absorbent pad used in a geriatric patient.

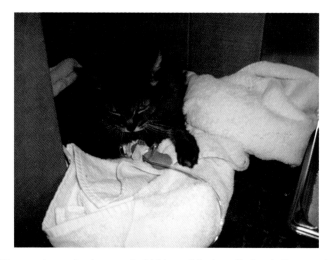

Figure 1.3 Many cats prefer to remain hidden while hospitalized. Here a simple cardboard box was used.

Noise and air quality

Ventilation, heating, and cooling are essential in maintaining patient husbandry in a clinical setting. Reducing noise is also imperative when it comes to patient comfort. Patients should be kept in a well-ventilated area. Many facilities have a smaller room with a door in which the vocal patients are kept. However, with this door being closed and several animals being excited and vocal, humidity and heat may result in unfavorable housing circumstances. Smaller patients usually need to be kept warm while larger, active, or brachycephalic patients may need to be kept in a cooler area. It is important to keep air circulating and unpleasant odors of either chemicals or excrement free from the patients' housing quarters.

Loud noises may startle patients suffering from anxiety, contributing to unfavorable psychological effects. When possible, loudly vocal patients disrupting ill, injured, or anxious patients should be removed from the area. In some cases, the vocal patient is suffering from anxiety or pain; these patients should be assessed for level of comfort and therapeutics administered as deemed appropriate.

Circadian rhythm

The circadian rhythm is a 24-hour cycle in which animals undergo biochemical and physiological processes such as sleeping and eating. Other processes affected by the circadian cycle include (but are not limited to) hormone production, digestion, and thermoregulation.

These processes may be influenced by the environment. For instance, the hormone melatonin peaks when the retina detects a dimmed light or darkness and is nearly absent during daylight hours. Melatonin is one of the hormones responsible for regulating the sleep-wake cycle; however, it is also thought to play a positive role in the immune systems' ability to fight infectious disease. Serotonin is the other main hormone regulating the sleep-wake cycle. Serotonin works opposite of melatonin, peaking during daylight hours and nearly absent during sleep. So while dim or dark light stimulates melatonin production and sleep, light stimulates serotonin production and the wake period of the circadian cycle. This becomes an important factor for patients receiving care in 24-hour facilities. When possible, lights should be dimmed during the overnight hours of hospitalization to keep this cycle regulated.

Infectious disease protocols

Patients suffering from infectious disease should be housed in a separate ward (isolation ward). Ideally, the isolation ward would be in a completely separate building; however, it is often located in a separate area of the practice with limited traffic. Having the isolation ward within the practice allows for personnel to observe and monitor these patients. Unfortunately, the result is a greater potential to spread disease throughout the practice and to ill or immunocompromised patients. Regardless, it is imperative to house infectious patients away from other patients to maintain disease control.

Isolation wards should include kennels, a sink, sanitation supplies, protective gowns, gloves, masks, shoe covers and caps for personnel to use, and an entire set of medical supplies, food dishes, and litter pans which remain in isolation. As a general rule, if something enters the isolation ward, it should not come out. This is not always possible, so it is imperative to thoroughly disinfect any supplies or instrumentation leaving the isolation ward. The fewer staff members entering and exiting the ward, the better chances that disease will not spread so long as proper procedures are followed. Traditionally, a separate bag for soiled laundry is kept and washed separately from other laundry. The disposable items such as shoe covers, gloves, and caps should be discarded prior to exiting the ward. Hands should be washed and a foot bath containing a disinfectant walked through while exiting. Once a patient leaves the isolation ward, it should undergo thorough sanitation. It is also recommended to have negative airflow into the isolation so when the entryways are opened, air moves into the ward, preventing airborne pathogens from escaping. As with any housing area, proper ventilation, humidity, and temperature control is essential (Fig. 1.4).

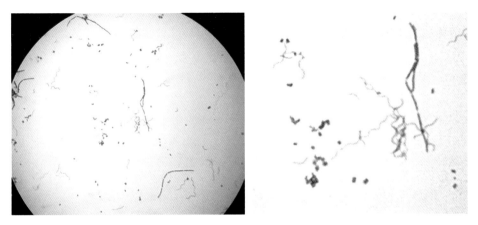

Figure 1.4 Microscopic view of mixed bacteria: cocci, bacilli, and spirochete.

Chapter references and further reading

S. Bateman (2008a) MRSA and MDA microbes: the OSU experience. International Veterinary Emergency and Critical Care Symposium.

S. Bateman (2008b) Infection control practices. International Veterinary Emergency and Critical Care Symposium.

R. Cheek (2009) What can you get from your pet? *Veterinary Technician the Complete Journal for the Veterinary Hospital Staff* **30**(6): 32-38.

A. Gordon (2009) You, the clinic, and methicillin-resistant staphylococcus. *Veterinary Technician the Complete Journal for the Veterinary Hospital Staff* **30**(1): 24-33.

L. Limon (2006) Nosocomial infections. *The National Association of Veterinary Technicians in America Journal* **Winter**: 29.

T. Mansueto (2004) Canine parvovirus infection- nursing is key. *Veterinary Technician the Complete Journal for the Veterinary Hospital Staff* **25**(11): 781-785.

J. Wilson (2007) Avoiding nosocomial infections. *The National Association of Veterinary Technicians in America Journal* **Summer**: 64-68.

Chapter 2
Considerations in Patient Management

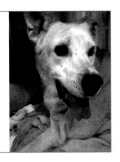

Hygiene and grooming

When veterinary patients are hospitalized, daily grooming and hygiene should be implemented by the veterinary staff. Grooming aids in cleanliness and ultimately has positive psychological as well as physical benefits for the patient. Many ill or injured patients are unable to or uninterested in grooming themselves. When this occurs, the veterinary nursing staff should ensure the patient is groomed daily or more frequently if needed (Fig. 2.1).

Patients should be brushed daily to help stimulate secretions from the sebaceous glands of the skin. Brushing will also help reduce matting and, in cats, reduce the risk of trichobezoars ("hair balls"). Brushing the patient will also serve as an opportunity to examine the skin for ectoparasites, wounds, petechiae or ecchymosis, jaundice, erythema, or any other abnormalities in the integumentary system. Patients should be brushed gently so as to prevent unnecessary pain. Brush strokes should be long and steady, reassuring for the patient. Most patients respond in a positive manner when brushed.

One of the most neglected aspects of veterinary patient care is instituting baths. Many recumbent or ill patients are soiled in their own feces, urine, or vomit while hospitalized. Too often the fur is patted dry and the application of hygiene spray applied. This leaves the skin vulnerable for infection. Any time a patient has soiled themselves, a bath or bathing of the local area is in order as long as the patient is stable enough to sustain the bath (Fig. 2.2). For patients with respiratory compromise or severe debilitation and anxiety, alternative methods can be used such as spot bathing with a bowl of warm soapy water, a bowl of clean water, and patting dry with a towel. The skin must be thoroughly cleansed to prevent scald and skin infection. The patient can be dried using a commercial grooming dryer or hair dryer. Care should be taken to ensure the heat setting will not cause thermal injury to the patient. While drying the patient, a hand can be placed between the warmed air and the patient; if the air is too hot for the hand

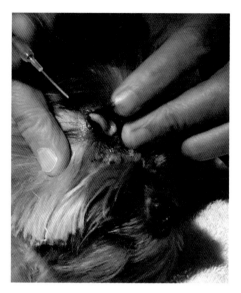

Figure 2.1 Smaller breeds prone to epiphora should have their tear secretions cleaned from hair and skin daily to prevent skin infection (lacrimal flush in a Yorkshire terrier suffering from dermatitis due to excessive tearing).

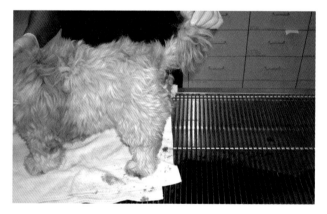

Figure 2.2 Preparing to bathe a dog with hemorrhagic gastroenteritis.

of the veterinary personnel, then it is most likely too hot for the patient and should be adjusted. Patients suffering from frequent vomiting and diarrhea, such as in parvovirus, generally benefit from a daily bath to rid the odor and cleanse the skin and fur as well as providing positive psychological benefits of bonding with the caregiver during this time. Patients suffering from emesis should have their mouths rinsed after an episode and, when necessary, hair clipped or cleansed and affected skin cleansed (Fig. 2.4).

Any time that excrement scald is suspected (Fig. 2.3), the area should be clipped free of hair, cleansed, and appropriate wound management implemented based on the stage of infection. It is recommended to use a size 10 clipper blade, being careful in prevention

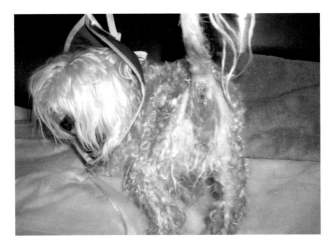

Figure 2.3 Excrement scald as a result of poor hygiene.

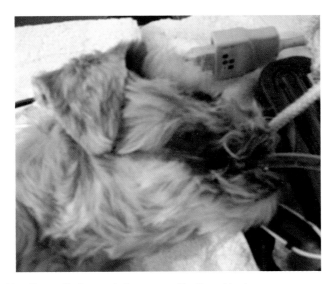

Figure 2.4 Vomitus soiled muzzle in an anesthetic patient.

abrasions. Hydrotherapy, vasoconstricting creams, and antibiotic ointments can be beneficial when treating dermal scald wounds. If the scald is due to urine leakage, a urinary catheter should be placed if patient and condition allows. Disposable absorbent pads can also be used to protect the skin by layering the pad in a manner that collects the material, sparing the patients' skin from exposure (Table 2.1, Figs. 2.5-2.9).

Nails should be clipped if they interfere with the patients' ability to ambulate. Older dogs tend to exercise less and have longer nails. Couple this with weakness, tile or slick floors, and anxiety and the result is generally an undesirable situation. Clipping the dogs' nails and laying blankets or towels may help the patient ambulate. Cats with longer, sharp nails should have a nail trim as this poses a safety risk for personnel. Care

Table 2.1 Preventing decubital ulcers and excrement scald

Task	Frequency	Rationale
Rotate patient position from lateral, sternal, semisternal, and opposing lateral recumbency	Every 2–4 hours	Altering positions will allow for perfusion of pressure points, helps prevent atelactasis
Provide thick, soft bedding, baby mattresses, pillows, pet beds, and so on	Bedding at all times, with rearrangement at each rotation. Bedding changed as frequently as necessary to provide a clean environment	Bedding will help prevent decubital ulcers by relieving pressure points. Areas of interest for padding include the shoulders, hips, elbows, lateral metatarsals, and lateral metacarpals
Full or partial bathing; sponge bathing	As frequently as needed to keep patient clean; any time the patient is soiled with urine, feces, vomit, food, and so on	Sponge bathing can be used to remove smaller amounts of debris, while partial and full baths should be given to ensure clean skin, preventing scald from the excrement
Towel or blow drying	After bathing; warm or cool air can be used with blow drying	Maintain euthermia, prevent moist dermatitis
Use of disposable pads	Change when soiled	Promote cleanliness in cases of diarrhea or emesis. Consider placing a urinary catheter and balancing fluid ins/outs with excessive urination
Use of over-the-counter (OTC) topical ointments an creams	After bathing	Diaper rash ointments will help protect the skin while hemorrhoid creams placed over areas at risk of decubital ulceration will cause vasoconstriction, reducing the inflammation
Implement physiotherapy	When applicable	Refer to section on physical therapy

should always be taken to prevent pain and hemorrhage by cutting the vessel or "quick" (Fig. 2.10).

Exercise and walks

Exercise and walks tend to be more pressing in dogs than in cats. Cats will often urinate and defecate in a litter box when they are in a kennel. Dogs, particularly those who are house trained, will tend to hold their bladder and bowels as long as they are kenneled.

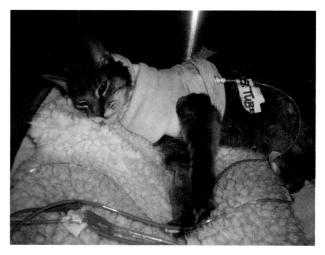

Figure 2.5   A recumbent patient, Maddie is resting in an elevated lateral recumbency on layers of bedding.

Dogs on higher fluid rates, those suffering from diarrhea or urinary infections and diabetics should be taken out for frequent walks. Care should be taken with patients suffering from anemia as overexertion and collapse is a possibility. Geriatric patients, patients suffering from osteoarthritis or recent trauma, fractures, or wounds should have slower, short walks on even ground. Patients with neurological conditions may need assisted walks, either being carried outside or supported with a towel or harness. Caution should always be displayed when a cardiac or respiratory patient is to be taken out for a walk, as too much exertion can prove to be fatal. Patients should be assessed for mental alertness, respiratory effort, ability to ambulate without excessive effort, and vital signs prior to a walk.

Exercise will promote coughing, clearing the airways in patients who have been housed in a kennel. During daylight hours, the sunshine will stimulate vitamin D production in the body, which aids in the proper function of the immune system. Sunlight also stimulates alertness and, in humans, has been shown to improve depression.

Although cats generally are not taken outside in the sunlight and fresh air, they too can receive the benefits of exercising. Cat toys can be used to stimulate the cat's mind and body while in the hospital. Additionally, a cat can be taken into an exam room and exposed to catnip (also called catmint or *Nepeta cataria*), which contains a chemical called nepetalactone, stimulating activity such as rolling, jumping, and frolicking in the herb. Not all cats will respond to catnip, and some will have an effect of calmness rather than activity.

Routine assessment and treatments

Veterinary patients who remain hospitalized for care generally have a treatment schedule or plan. Patients should be observed routinely, with vital signs assessed and documented as often as necessary, depending on the nature of the condition. It is not

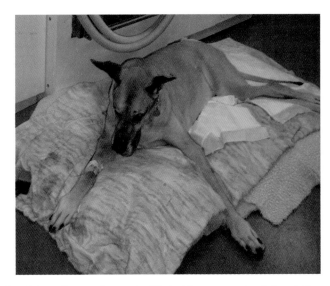

Figure 2.6   Semisternal recumbency instituted in a recumbent Great Dane.

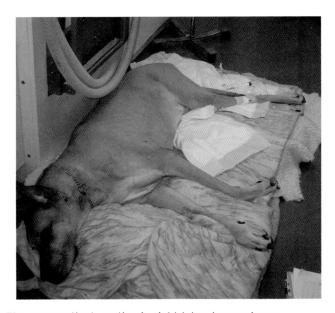

Figure 2.7   The same patient, resting in right lateral recumbency.

uncommon for patients in the ICU to have continuous monitoring 24 hours a day until status has improved.

The veterinarian or technician usually creates the treatment plan, indicating a set schedule for obtaining vital signs, administering medications, and walking outside. Veterinary nursing applications should also be implemented. For instance, the recumbent patient should have positional changes at least every 4 hours, feeding should be instituted, bedding changed, and fluid balances calculated. Unfortunately, when these

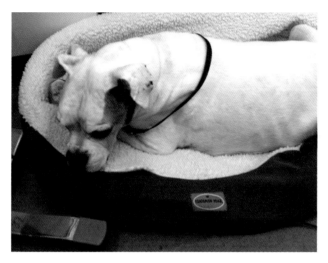

Figure 2.8 The use of a commercial pet bed in an anemic patient receiving a whole blood transfusion.

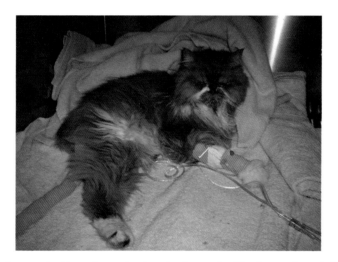

Figure 2.9 Demonstration of poor husbandry in a cat with glomerulonephritis: vomitus visible on fur surrounding chin; vomitus and blood are evident on bedding; and edematous extremities, which would benefit from massage and range-of-motion exercises. The tail, however, is wrapped for hygiene.

tasks are not definitively outlined in a treatment schedule, they may become overlooked when they should ultimately be standard practices in nursing care (Fig. 2.11).

Another aspect of patient assessment includes the pairing of staff members to patients. When a staff member has been caring for a particular patient, they may be likely to notice subtle changes, such as respiratory pattern changes or signs of pain. Additionally, a bond is established and the patient then knows the individual and may feel more comfortable. An alternative method of monitoring includes having veterinary

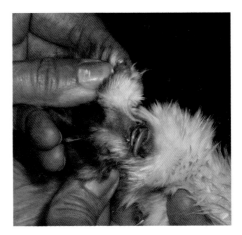

Figure 2.10 Overgrown nail in a cat which has penetrated through and exited surrounding tissue.

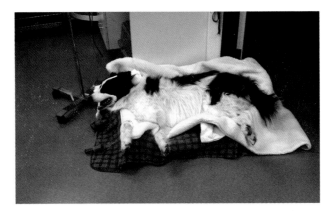

Figure 2.11 A recumbent patient placed in clear view rather than in a run or kennel to optimize husbandry and needs.

personnel rotate between patients. This technique can bring a fresh assessment, notice trend changes, or can shed light to needs that may improve the well-being of the patient.

Pain assessment

Recognizing signs of pain and advocating pain management is a paramount element of patient care. It is well recognized that patients, both veterinary and human, suffer from longer hospital stays, greater complications, and increased mortality when allowed to remain in uncontrolled pain. It is assumed that any condition which may cause pain to humans would indeed cause pain to animals as well. The first step to pain management is clinically recognizing signs of pain.

From a physiological standpoint, common vital sign parameters will reflect the stimulation of the sympathetic nervous system when an animal is in pain. Most commonly noted are increased heart rate and blood pressure, increased respiratory rate, and mydriasis. Although these are physiological effects of pain, it is important to note that

Table 2.2 Recognition of pain

Physiological affects	• Increased heart rate and blood pressure; peripheral vasoconstriction with possible cool extremities; prolonged capillary refill time (CRT) • Tachypnea or panting • Ptyalism, inappetance, vomiting, diarrhea, or constipation • Muscle fasciculations, weakness, difficult or reluctant ambulation • Neutrophilia, lymphocytosis, hyperglycemia, and polycythemia; elevated cortisol and catecholamine
Behavioral affects	• Vocality • Pacing or lack of mobility • Aggression or apprehension • Inadequate or absent grooming • Lack of appetite
Localized areas	• Eye: squinting, rubbing eye • Ear: shaking head, rubbing or scratching ears • Mouth: ptyalism, cautious eating or drinking • Musculoskeletal: ataxia or other altered gait, reluctant when ambulating, dysuria, stranguria, or tenesmus • Abdomen: splinting, postural changes ("hunched back"), anorexia, or vomiting • Thorax: respiratory rate and pattern changes, orthopnea, reluctant ambulation, vocality • Extremities: nonweight bearing, licking, biting or chewing • Perianal: licking, chewing, tenesmus, or scooting

Table 2.3 Physiological processes of pain

Transduction	Translation of stimuli into electrical activity
Transmission	Movement of the impulses to spinal cord
Modulation	Movement of impulses from spinal cord to brain
Perception	The brain recognizing the pain

fear, stress, and anxiety can also stimulate the "fight-or-flight" response with similar clinical responses.

Behavioral changes, in addition to physiological parameters, will aid in the assessment of pain. The behavioral response to pain may vary not only between dogs and cats, but also between breeds. Some breeds tend to have a high tolerance to pain while others may not. There is not an established standard veterinary pain scale; however, the majority of pain scales in use are based on behavioral characteristics for a specific species. Some behavioral changes in response to pain are listed in Table 2.2.

Veterinary technicians work more closely with the patients so it is only practical and good reasoning for the veterinary support staff to be advocates of pain management. There are many techniques to providing pain management, including (but not limited to) the application of physical therapy, the use of narcotics and anti-inflammatory drugs, and the administration of local anesthetics or regional nerve blocks. A patient with a chest tube may benefit from a local anesthetic administered into the thorax (via the chest tube), while a patient with pitting edema would benefit from physical therapy applications (Table 2.3).

Psychological health

Hospitalized patients require certain emotional needs as well as physical environmental needs to be met. Many times these patients are painful, scared, nervous, and uncomfortable. It may bring comfort to the pet to have blankets, beds, or toys from home as well as receiving visits from family members. Occasionally, when owner visits end, some patients go through a period of extreme anxiety. In those cases, visits may not be in the best interest of the patient (Figs. 2.12 and 2.13).

Patients should receive tender loving care while hospitalized. Talking to them during treatments and assessments may help ease the patient and bridge the bond with the

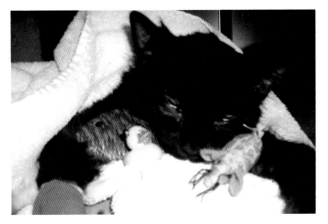

Figure 2.12 Post-operative pain management: B.B. is recovering with his own (catnip) toys.

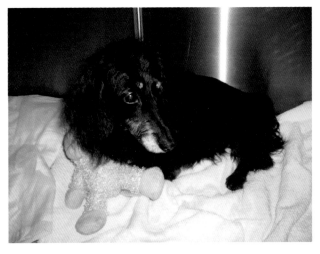

Figure 2.13 A nervous dachshund has been provided toys from his home to help ease his hospital stay.

caregiver. Petting the patient with long, firm strokes can help reduce anxiety and discomfort. Care should be taken to minimize loud or sudden movements which may startle the patients. Some patients may also benefit from a more secluded area of housing. For instance, if a nervous or vocal dog is residing next to an ill cat, both patients may benefit from the vocal patient being moved to a more secluded, calm area of the practice. In extreme cases of anxiety, sedatives may be warranted to allow the patient (and other hospitalized patients) to rest peacefully.

Care for the recumbent patient

Recumbency can occur in several disease states, from a neurological condition to critical illness. Nonambulatory patients should be provided with soft bedding, with attention to pressure points such as shoulders, stifles, and hips. These areas are prone to developing decubital ulcers or "bed sores." This serious and sometimes fatal condition is a reflection of nursing care provided. Decubital ulcers can be preventable and efforts should always be made in anticipation of the occurrence. Proactive measures include the use of blankets, crib mattresses, pet water beds, and pressure-relieving foam material. Stockinet material can be rolled up into a "donut" to prevent pressure in areas such as the elbow or hip. Decubital ulcers occur when there is either a lack of circulation or reperfusion injury to the region. The area becomes red and painful as cell death occurs. If the wounds break open, the risk of infection and subsequent sepsis is a serious one as it may be the be-all and end-all to the already immunocompromised patient (Fig. 2.14, Table 2.4).

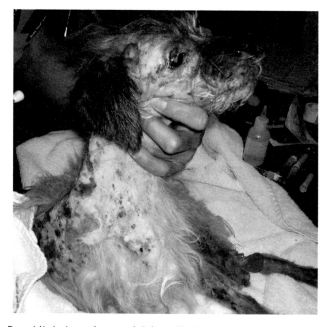

Figure 2.14 Decubital ulcers in a geriatric patient.

Table 2.4 Decubitus ulcer classification

Stages	Description	Nursing interventions
Stage one	Superficial, nonblanchable erythema	Astute recognition and therapeutics: relieve pressure using devices such as cushions, improve patient nutrition and hydration, implement comprehensive wound evaluations
Stage two	Epidermis and dermis injury, partial thickness loss, ruptured or intact abrasion noted	Continue measures to alleviate pressure, clean wounds and cover open wounds. Wound care may range from wet-to-dry bandages to hydrotherapy for debridement or the application of hydrocolloid dressing or hyperbaric oxygen (topical or chamber therapy)
Stage three	Injury to the subcutaneous layer, full thickness loss	Maintain and potentially improve previous therapeutics such as nutrition and fluid therapy; consider low laser therapy
Stage four	Injury extends to muscle, joint capsule, or bone	Consider advocating surgical intervention (closure, flap, or graft)

Recumbent patients should be rotated at least every 2–4 hours, moving from lateral to sternal or semisternal recumbency as permitted by patient needs and condition. Positional changes will not only help prevent pressure sores, it will also help prevent atelactasis.

Finally, recumbent patients without indwelling urinary catheters require assistance with micturition. In efforts to promote natural urination, recumbent dogs may be carried outside and assisted while cats may be assisted in a litter box. If the patients' physical state does not allow for this technique, or if the technique is unsuccessful, then manual expressing of the bladder is indicated. The bladder should be palpated for size, thickness, and ease of manual voiding. With manual expressing of the bladder, attention to the urine quantity and quality (gross examination) should be evaluated. Recumbent patients are often unable to fully void the bladder of urine. This remaining urine collects and bladder infections ensue, resulting in a classic strong odor (Fig. 2.15).

Detecting abnormalities

The ability to detect abnormalities in the veterinary patient is one of great skill. Understanding first what is normal for the patient, for the condition, for the therapeutics administered, and then recognizing when those observations have deviated, is a talent in itself. With experience and continuous learning, specific characteristics of conditions and symptoms of conditions will become more easily recognized.

Documentation is essential when it comes to detecting abnormalities. Documentation should include (but is not limited to) alertness, vital sign notation, fluid balances, heart and lung sounds, positional arrangement, behavioral observations, and nutritional status. Each change or abnormality should be documented, regardless how casual, meager, or inappreciable it may seem at the time. It is imperative that veterinary nursing staff caring for patients not only understand the anatomy, physiology, and pathophysiology of their patients' condition, but also recognize changes and prepare for (and hopefully prevent) the next step of the disease process. Proactive nursing care involves critical thinking skills, preventing a patient from deteriorating, and ultimately improving the health and well-being of the patient (Figs. 2.16–2.19).

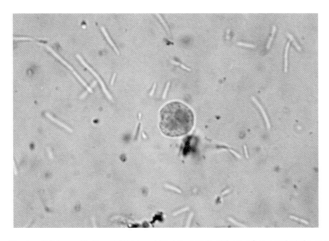

Figure 2.15 *Escherichia coli* (bacilli) in a bladder infection of a geriatric patient. A white blood cell (WBC, center) is also present.

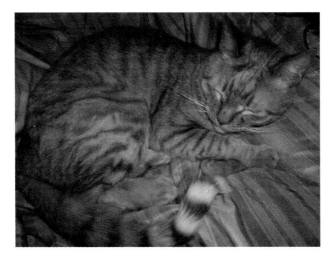

Figure 2.16 Tommy resting comfortably (fibrosarcoma in the left pelvic limb).

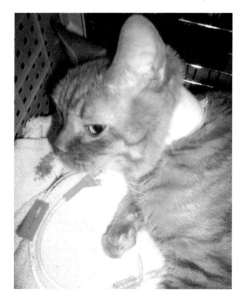

Figure 2.17 The previous patient, Tommy, suffering from post-operative pain (amputation). Note the change in expression, particularly the eyes.

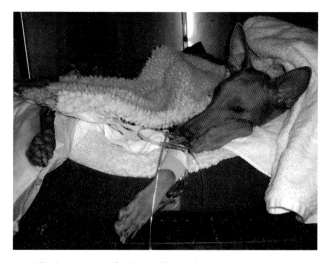

Figure 2.18 A vestibular yet comfortable Pharaoh Hound.

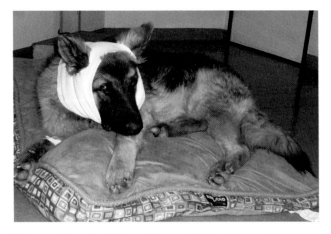

Figure 2.19 A German Shepherd Dog with a painful neck wound.

Chapter references and further reading

A. Gottlieb (2002) Analgesic options for managing pain in cats and dogs. *Veterinary Technician the Complete Journal for the Veterinary Hospital Staff* **23**(10): 638-645.

A. Gottlieb (2009) No pain plenty of gain. *Veterinary Technician the Complete Journal for the Veterinary Hospital Staff* **30**(3): 16-22.

P. Hellyer (2003) Introduction to pain management. *The National Association of Veterinary Technicians in America Journal* **Spring**: 54-58.

J. Kerr (2008) Unique feline monitoring and management techniques. International Veterinary Emergency and Critical Care Symposium.

H. Madsen (2005) Perioperative pain management. *Veterinary Technician the Complete Journal for the Veterinary Hospital Staff* **26**(5): 359-368.

J. Mott (2004) Ethical decision making: dealing with dilemmas and improving patient care. *Veterinary Technician the Complete Journal for the Veterinary Hospital Staff* **25**(2): 126-131.

M. Schaer (2003) Clinical pearls in intensive and critical care I and II. Western Veterinary Conference.

N. Schaffran (1998) Pain in critically ill small animals: ethical aspects. *Veterinary Technician the Complete Journal for the Veterinary Hospital Staff* **19**(5): 349-353.

N. Schaffran (2002) Common protocols for pain management. *Veterinary Technician the Complete Journal for the Veterinary Hospital Staff* **23**(12): 748-753.

N. Schaffran (2003) Pain relief as a practice standard. *Veterinary Technician the Complete Journal for the Veterinary Hospital Staff* **24**(1): 36-38.

R. Sereno (2005) Pain management for cancer patients. *The National Association of Veterinary Technicians in America Journal* **Winter**: 45-50.

Chapter 3
Patient Exam and Assessments

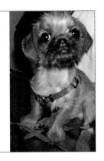

Obtaining and interpreting vital signs

Obtaining, interpreting, and assessing vital sign parameters of a patient is generally an involved process. The patient should undergo a primary survey, noting any changes in mentation, posture, pain level, urination, or defecation. The basic parameters to be measured include the temperature, heart rate, pulse quality, respiration, mucous membrane (MM) assessment, and capillary refill time (CRT). By obtaining and documenting the findings in these measurements, abnormalities in body systems can be detected. This chapter will cover the general guidelines and assessment of vital signs. Pathophysiology, detailed monitoring, and interventions can be found in the comprehensive areas of focus section.

Temperature

The temperature can be measured using aural, axillary, toe web, esophageal, or rectal routes, with the latter being most reliable. Temperatures obtained via the aural (ear) route can be used in patients with rectal abnormalities; however, with the L-shaped ear canal, results may not be accurate. The axillary (under forearm) method can be used with fractious patients; however, obtaining a temperature via this route takes a minimum of 4 minutes for accuracy (using a mercury thermometer) and the results can be falsely elevated. Using the toe web method is best when used in conjunction with a rectal temperature reading. A difference greater than 7° can indicate poor perfusion. Esophageal thermometers have been incorporated into most multiparameter surgical monitors and are generally reserved for anesthetized patients. Obtaining the temperature rectally is the most common and preferred approach. This method is the most accurate and reliable. The rectal method should be used with caution when the animal has sustained injury (or surgery) in the rectal area.

Clinical Small Animal Care: Promoting Patient Health through Preventative Nursing, First Edition. Kimm Wuestenberg.
© 2012 John Wiley & Sons, Inc. Published 2012 by John Wiley & Sons, Inc.

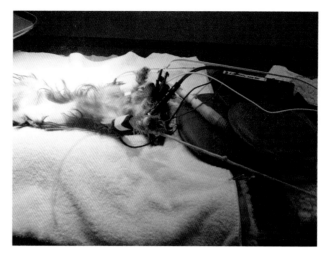

Figure 3.1 Warming techniques including circulating water blanket, IV fluid warmer, and warming the airway.

An animal's body temperature can be an indicator of several conditions. Stress can cause a slightly elevated temperature, but other conditions such as infection, heat exhaustion, seizures, and certain toxicities (i.e., toad toxicity) can also cause an elevation. Hypothermia can be caused by conditions such as shock, metabolic crisis, environmental conditions, and anesthesia.

When a patients' body temperature is significantly out of normal range, it is important that the animal's temperature is not adjusted too quickly. If there is a rapid change in temperature, it could cause serious problems for the patient. For instance, rapid cooling can contribute to a severe coagulopathy such as disseminated intravascular coagulation. Rapid heating can cause vasodilatation, which may result in lowering the blood pressure of the animal. If external heating or cooling sources are necessary, the temperature should be adjusted slowly and ceased once the animal is within 2° of normalcy. This is to prevent heating and cooling methods from exceeding the ideal temperature, as the body will continue to heat (or cool) once external sources have ceased (Figs. 3.1 and 3.2).

Pulse and heart rate

The pulse represents the left ventricular force or delivery of blood to the body. When assessing the pulse, the heart should also be included in the survey. Each pulse should represent one cardiac cycle; therefore, with each heartbeat, there should be a pulse that follows. However, there are times when there is not a palpable pulse detected with every heartbeat; this is referred to as a pulse deficit. Pulse deficits can occur in patients with (but not limited to) primary cardiac disease, splenic masses, gastric dilatation and volvulus, pain, and hypoxia, among numerous other conditions. It is important to listen to the heart while palpating pulses to confirm synchronicity of the two processes.

The most common areas to palpate pulses are the femoral artery, the axillary artery, and the dorsal metatarsal artery. The strength or amount of force (quality) of the pulse

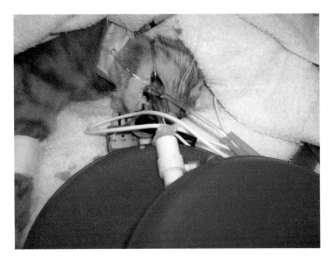

Figure 3.2 Warming the patient airway.

Table 3.1 Cardiac murmurs

Grade (intensity)	Description
I/VI	Barely audible, soft murmur audible after few minutes of auscultation
II/VI	Heard immediately, soft murmur localized to one valve area
III/VI	Immediately audible, moderate intensity, noted at more than one location
IV/VI	Moderate to loud intensity, but no precordial thrill
V/VI	Loud intensity, palpable precordial thrill present
VI/VI	Loud intensity, precordial thrill, audible with stethoscope away from thoracic wall

should be observed. If the pulse is very strong or bounding, it can be indicative of pain, anxiety, or hypertension. If the pulse quality is weak or poor, it can be indicative of poor perfusion, low blood pressure, or end-stage disease.

The heart should be auscultated and observed for the presence of heart murmurs, arrhythmias, bradycardia, tachycardia, or muffled sounds. Some animals develop murmurs during illness, in which the murmur goes away once the patient has recovered. A murmur will have a "whoosh" sound instead of clear, distinct heart sounds the normal healthy cardiac patient has. There are different degrees of murmurs. Muffled or absent heart sounds can be associated with fluid in the thoracic cavity, particularly the pericardium (Table 3.1).

Normal Heart Rates:

Small dog: 100–160 beats per minute
Medium to large dogs: 60–100 beats per minute
Cats: 110–240 beats per minute

Respiration rate and pattern

Respiratory rate and pattern is assessed by auscultating the lungs and observing the pattern. Abnormal respiratory patterns can oftentimes help determine the area of the respiratory system affected. An increase in inspiratory effort, marked with open mouth breathing or gasping motions, usually corresponds to an upper airway condition. There may be an audible sound (stridor or stertor) with respirations when there is upper airway involvement.

An increase in expiratory effort, marked with an increase in abdominal effort or contracting, is indicative of a lower respiratory condition. Some conditions associated with abdominal breathing and expiratory distresses are right-sided heart disease, diaphragmatic hernia, acute respiratory distress syndrome (ARDS), and pneumonia. Certain conditions may have little or no inspiratory or expiratory effort; however, the animal may still be in respiratory distress. Watching the pattern is important. Shallow, fast respirations are associated with conditions such as a pneumothorax and a pleural effusion. Animals with asthma, pulmonary contusions, or pulmonary thromboembolism (PTE) can appear to have severe inspiratory and expiratory effort at the same time, along with open mouth breathing and tachypnea.

When auscultating the lungs, breath sounds should be heard for both inspiration and expiration. As with the heart, it is a good idea to listen to normal, healthy lungs of several animals so abnormal breath sounds can be recognized. Common abnormal sounds that may be noted are wheezes (whistling) and crepitant and crackling rales (popping or bubbling sounds). Wheezes are associated with bronchitis and asthma. Crepitant and crackling rales are associated with fluid in the lungs (pneumonia, pulmonary edema, near drowning, etc.). It is important to note which side of the thorax the sounds were observed, and whether it was the cranial (toward the head) or caudal (toward the tail) area of the thorax, and whether the sounds were heard upon inspiration or expiration.

Normal Respirations:

Dog: 8-20 breaths per minute
Cat: 8-30 breaths per minute

MM and CRT

In addition to the TPR, the pet's MMs and CRT should be assessed. The gingival MMs are primarily observed; however, the conjunctiva or perianal region can be used for assessment. MMs are normally a coral pink color. Patients with pigmented gingival may be difficult to assess. Pale MMs can be an indicator for conditions such as shock, anemia, hypothermia, or pain. Bright red, injected, or hyperemic MMs can indicate conditions such as septic shock, hypertension, or toxicosis. MMs displaying a brown color can indicate acetaminophen or carbon monoxide toxicosis while yellowing, or icterus, typically accompanies conditions of the hepatobiliary system. Cyanosis is often observed in patients suffering from respiratory distress. Cyanosis is usually one of the last indicators that the pet is hypoxic.

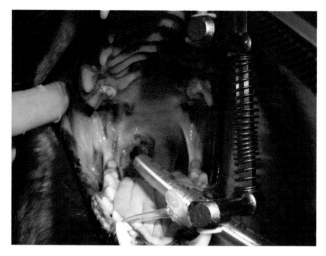

Figure 3.3 Normal pink MM color in a dog with oral squamous cell carcinoma.

The MM should also be assessed for moisture. Tacky (dry/sticky) MMs can be indicative of dehydration, whereas moist MMs can be associated with toxins, nausea, or overhydration.

The CRT is obtained by pressing on an area of the gingival MMs. The area will become blanched, then fill with color again. The total time this should take is 1-2 seconds. A CRT less than 1 second can indicate a hyperdynamic state, whereas a CRT longer than 3 seconds can indicate poor perfusion. The CRT can be utilized as a quick reference of the patients' perfusion. A measurement of blood pressure should be performed if the CRT is either rapid or delayed (Figs. 3.3–3.6).

Patient monitoring equipment

Although there are many useful machines and monitoring units readily available in most veterinary settings, the most important one is the veterinary nursing staff. With that being said, utilizing the available instrumentation will help in better assessment and perhaps verification of clinical findings by the veterinary personnel. Most commonly used devices are blood pressure monitors, pulse oximetry machines, electrocardiographs, and capnographs. These machines are useful in both perioperative nursing and in monitoring the ill or injured patient.

Blood pressure monitoring

Blood pressure can be measured using direct or indirect means. Direct blood pressure monitoring is invasive and requires the use of an arterial catheter. Indirect blood pressure monitoring is obtained by using either an ultrasound flow detector (Doppler) or an oscillometer (typically part of multiparameter monitoring machines). Blood pressure

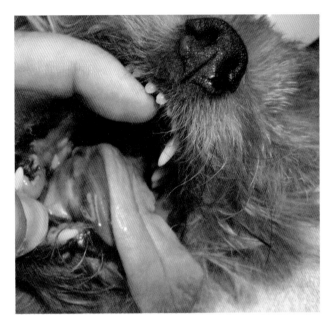

Figure 3.4 Cyanotic MM color in a dog suffering asphyxia due to rattlesnake envenomation.

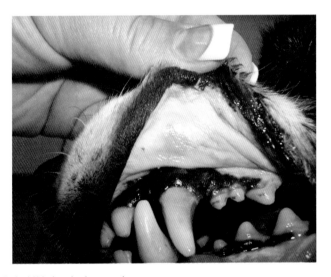

Figure 3.5 Pale MM due to hemorrhage.

should be monitored in any patient with cardiovascular instability or any patient undergoing anesthetic or surgical procedures. Measurements are commonly taken by using the extremities, though the tail can be used, and in instances of cardiopulmonary arrest, the Doppler transducer may be placed on the cornea to detect blood flow to the brain.

The normal blood pressure is 120/80, with a mean arterial pressure (MAP) of 70-110. The first number (120) is the systolic pressure, the pressure in the arteries during the

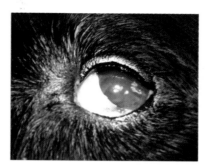

Figure 3.6 Pallor of third eyelid with concurrent hyphema of the eye in a coagulaopathy.

contractual phase of the cardiac cycle. The second number (80) represents the diastolic pressure in the arteries during the relaxing or refilling phase of the cycle. The MAP is the time-averaged value of pressure in the arteries. To manually calculate the MAP, the formula $S + (2 \times D)/3$ can be used. Oscillometric blood pressure machines typically calculate the MAP so this formula is more often used when using the Doppler to obtain blood pressure values.

Blood pressure cuff selection can greatly influence readings. A cuff that is too small may cause a falsely elevated blood pressure while a large cuff can falsely lower the reading. The cuff width should be approximately 40% of the limb circumference. A quick estimation can be made by choosing a cuff with the same height as the width of the portion of the extremity to be used. The bladder of the cuff should be placed over the artery. The cuff should be completely deflated in between measurements to prevent inaccurate readings (Figs. 3.7–3.9).

Pulse oximetry

The pulse oximeter is a machine that gives a percentage of oxygen saturation in the body. Most machines give an audible pulse rate with tone sounds corresponding to the level (or percentage) of oxygenation and a visual pulse wave displaying a measurement of pulse strength. The pulse oximeter is an indicator, but not necessarily a true measurement of oxygenation and delivery. The value obtained is strictly limited to the vessel in which the values were obtained. For instance, a pulse oximetry reading obtained from the tongue does not necessarily represent the oxygen saturation in a particular extremity. The normal oxygen saturation reading is 95% or greater.

Oxygen content should also be assessed when evaluating oxygen saturation. The normal oxygen content is 20 mL/dL, with an acceptable range of 17–24 mL/dL. The value of a patients' oxygen content can be obtained by using this simple formula:

$$\text{Oxygen content} = 1.36 \times \text{saturation} \times (\text{packed cell volume}/3).$$

This formula is important to incorporate into oxygenation status, as a severely anemic patient can have a saturation of 96%, but may have dangerously low oxygen content since oxygen is transported via hemoglobin molecules within a red blood cell.

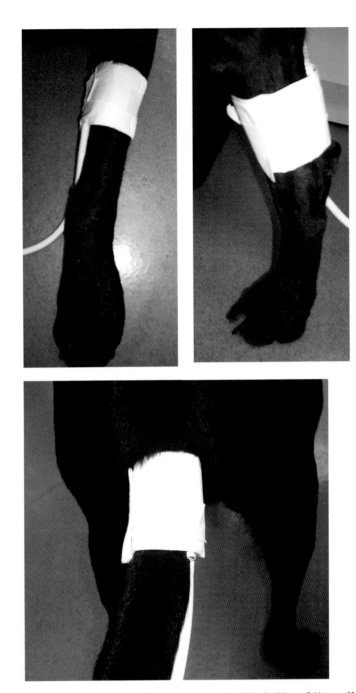

Figures 3.7-3.9 Blood pressure cuff placement; note the ladder of the cuff is on the medial aspect of the limbs and the ventral aspect of the tail.

It should be noted that while pulse oximetry provides a percentage of oxygen saturation within a vessel, it does not measure or provide information about the delivery of oxygen to other tissues in the body (perfusion).

Capnography

The capnograph is a useful tool when assessing ventilation when a patient has an endotracheal tube in place. The capnograph measures carbon dioxide in the respiratory cycle by taking the measurements from the remaining air at the end of the endotracheal tube. The capnograph can help detect poor pulmonary perfusion resulting from instances such as kinks in an endotracheal tube, esophageal intubation, a malfunctioning anesthesia machine, and the occurrence of apnea.

There are four phases in the capnogram cycle. Phase I is an inspiratory baseline and should have a value of zero as the patient should not be inhaling carbon dioxide. Phase II is usually a steep climb, representing the expiratory upstroke when carbon dioxide first meets the sensor just as exhalation begins. Phase III of the capnogram represents the exhaled carbon dioxide as a plateau. The peak of this plateau is referred to as the end-title carbon dioxide as it is the last phase of expiration. Phase IV is the inspiratory downstroke marking the beginning of the inspiratory phase with a significant reduction in carbon dioxide as oxygen is entering the airway.

Electrocardiography (ECG)

Electrocardiograms are commonly used intraoperatively as a tool for cardiac monitoring. From intraoperative care, the use of electrocardiograms can expand to monitoring critically ill or injured patients in addition to any patient displaying pulse deficits, bradycardia, tachycardia, or auscultated dysrhythmias.

The electrocardiogram is a visual representation of the electrical activity of the heart. The amplitude of the complex shows the amount of electrical activity and the duration shows the length of time involved with the conduction. Each (normal) complex is made of up of the P wave, the QRS complex, and the T wave.

The P wave occurs from depolarization (contraction) of the right and left atria and is the first wave in the complex. The Q, R, and S waves make up the QRS complex, which represents ventricular depolarization (contraction). The T wave is the last wave of the complex and occurs when both ventricles repolarize (relaxation phase).

In addition to the waves conducted, the segment intervals are also evaluated. The PR interval marks the time from atrial depolarization to ventricular depolarization. The QT interval marks the time in which ventricular depolarization and repolarization occur. Lastly, the ST segment is the time between the ending of ventricular depolarization and the beginning of ventricular repolarization (Table 3.2, Fig. 3.10).

Thermoregulation

Induced hypothermia has been used in medicine since the time of Hippocrates and is still currently used in modern medicine in both ischemic and nonischemic conditions. Hypothermia has shown to be beneficial in treatment of brain injury, cardiac arrest,

Table 3.2 Determining heart rate and rhythm using the electrocardiogram

Obtaining the heart rate:

RR interval (1500 or 3000) method:

50 mm/s: count the number of small boxes between two R waves and divide by 3000 to get beats per minute.

25 mm/s: count the number of small boxes between two R waves and divide by 1500 to get beats per minute.

Sequence method:

Count the number of R waves (or P waves) in a 6-second strip and multiply by 10.

Observing the heart rhythm:

PR interval:

The time from the signal in the sinoatrial (SA) node, which depolarizes the atria to the moment the signal crosses into the ventricle, usually through the atrioventricular (AV) node.

QRS segment:

The time it takes to depolarize the ventricles

QT interval:

The onset of ventricular depolarization to the completion of ventricular repolarization.

Normal parameters

Description	Canine (seconds)	Canine (mV)	Feline (seconds)	Feline (mV)
P wave	0.04	0.4	0.04	0.4
PR interval	0.06–0.13		0.05–0.09	
QRS complex	0.05–0.06 (max)	2.5–3.0 (max)	0.04 (max)	0.9 (max)
QT interval	0.15–0.25		0.12–0.18	
ST segment		0.2 (max)		0.1 (max)
T wave		<25% of R wave height		<25% of R wave height

stroke, and status epilepticus. While some patients may benefit from induced hypothermia, an unplanned hypothermia may contribute to prolonged recovery, impaired blood clotting, altered drug metabolism, surgical site infection, and even cardiovascular ischemia.

Human studies have shown that maintaining euthermia in perioperative patients contributes to patient comfort and satisfaction. Veterinary patients undergoing an anesthetic procedure should have vital signs obtained prior to anesthesia and vigilantly watched for hypothermia throughout the procedure. Additionally, preventative measures should be taken in anticipation of hypothermia by implementing warming techniques in patients at risk. Surgical and anesthetic patients may benefit from preoperative,

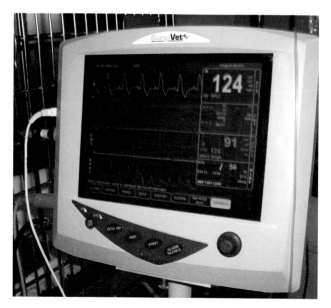

Figure 3.10 Multiparameter monitor displaying left bundle branch block (ECG) and low oxygen percentage (pulse oximeter).

intraoperative, and postoperative warming according to human anesthetic nursing literature.

It is well recognized that anesthetic agents and opiates contribute to hypothermia. Patients suffering from cardiovascular impairment consequently suffer reduced blood flow to vital organs such as the kidneys, which receive approximately 25% of cardiac output, and the liver, which receives approximately 33% of cardiac output. Thermoregulatory vasoconstriction may contribute to additional loss of blood flow to tissues and vital organs as well as creating venous stasis. Hypothermia-induced vasoconstriction can mask a hypovolemic state, and when rewarming techniques are implemented in this scenario, hypotension, circulatory shock, and *circulus vitiosus* may ensue.

In addition to cardiovascular effects, hypothermia has shown to directly affect the immune system and coagulation, which may contribute to increased blood loss and need for blood transfusions. Perioperative hypothermia has been associated with wound infections, blood loss, myocardial ischemia, pain, prolonged recovery time, and cardiac disturbances. In the emergency or intensive care unit (ICU) setting, hypothermia can contribute to poor oxygenation when dysfunctional blood flow is present, prolong the healing of traumatic or chronic wounds, and contribute to a longer hospital stay, placing the patient at risk for nosocomial infections.

The veterinary nursing staff should institute guidelines for hypothermic and anesthetic patients as anesthesia increases the risk of hypothermia. Providing a protocol for patient thermal monitoring will benefit the patient as well as designate responsibility and accountability for the patients' thermoregulation. A guideline for the use of thermal interventions may also be helpful since a variety of warming sources are available in most practices.

External heating applications include the use of commercially available tools such as forced-air warming systems, heating pads that may or may not include water circulation, heat lamps, and heating disks. Alternatively, warming applications commonly made in the clinic include the use of hair dryers, rice bags, and warm fluid bags or bottles.

A great risk of external heating is the induction of thermal injury to the patients' dermis. Any time external heating is applied to a patient special care must be taken to prevent burns. Creating a barrier between the patient and the heat source will help prevent such injury. A towel may used as a barrier with hot water bottles, and when a hairdryer is used, a hand should be placed between the patient and hairdryer to monitor for excessive heat. Warm-air units are usually low risk when it comes to thermal injury.

It is important to understand that many external heating sources are warming just that, the external body, and not necessarily warming the patents' core. Internal warming is an excellent way to help promote euthermia. Internal warming can be implemented by the use of warmed intravenous (IV) fluids, warmed lavage fluids during surgical procedures, and warmed inhaled oxygen and gases. In some cases, warm water enemas can be used as a warming technique. Although internal warming is effective, it cannot be depended on alone and should be used in conjunction with other methods of warming.

There are circumstances in medicine where hypothermia is a desired state; however, it is important to understand the effects of hypothermia on patients with inadvertent hypothermia and recognize those at risk for hypothermia. Being proactive in thermoregulation has shown to improve patient comfort, healing, and recovery time. The benefits of patient warming greatly outweigh the severe consequences that have been associated with hypothermia. It is essential that veterinary personnel appreciate the importance of thermoregulation and help promote guidelines and protocols for patients at risk for hypothermia (Figs. 3.11-3.13, Tables 3.3 and 3.4).

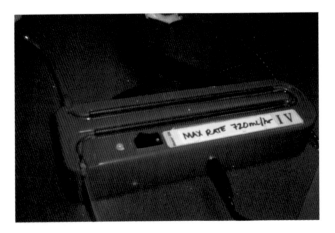

Figure 3.11 Fluid warmer.

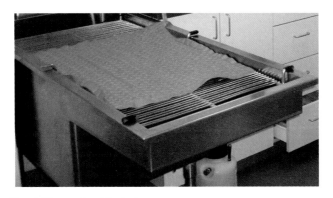

Figure 3.12 Circulating water blanket.

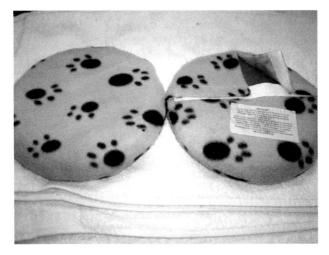

Figure 3.13 Warming disks.

Table 3.3 Vital sign parameters

Heart rate (beats per minute)	Small dog: 100–160 beats per minute
	Medium to large dogs: 60–100 beats per minute
	Cats: 110–240 beats per minute
Respirations (breaths per minute)	Dog: 8–20 breaths per minute
	Cat: 8–30 breaths per minute
Temperature	100.5–102.5°F
MM	Coral pink, moist
CRT	<2 seconds
Blood pressure	120/80
	MAP 70–110
	Central venous pressure (CVP) 0–5 mmH$_2$O

Table 3.4 Patient monitoring flow sheet

Date:		Patient:				Owner:		
Condition:						Dr:		Tech:

Meds	Strength	Dose	Route	Time	Initials	DNR:	Wt:
						IVC	
						Special Concerns:	
							Fluid Type:
							Rate:
							Total Volume:
						Monitoring:	
						Pulse Ox ☐ Bp ☐	
						ECG ☐ Temp ☐	
						Capnograph ☐ Other: ☐	

Time:								
Fluids In								
Fluids Out								
O₂ Rate								
Pulse Ox:								
Temp:								
190								
180								
170								
160								
150								
140								
130								
120								
110								
100								
90								
80								
70								
60								
50								
40								
30								
20								
10								
0								

HR ●	Notes:
RR ○	
Sys △	
Dias ▽	
MAP ☆	

DNR, do not resuscitate; Wt, weight; IVC, intravenous catheter; Pulse Ox, pulse oximetry; ECG, electrocardiography; BP, blood pressure; Temp, temperature; HR, heart rate; RR, respiratory rate; Sys, systolic; Dias, diastolic; Post-Op, postoperative.

Chapter references and further reading

B. Bulmer (2006) Performing a cardiovascular physical examination. *Veterinary Medicine* **January**.

R. Gfeller, et al. (1994) Physical exam checklist for pets. Veterinary Information Network.

E. Mazzaferro (2003) Respiratory system evaluation and monitoring. American Animal Hospital Association Scientific Program.

R. Pottie, et al (2007) Effect of hypothermia on recovery from general anesthesia in the dog. *Australian Veterinary Journal* **85**(4).

H. Ruess-Lamky (2008) Anesthetic monitors: understanding their use and limitations. *The National Association of Veterinary Technicians in America Journal* **Spring**: 60-67.

M. Tefend (2004) Hemodynamic monitoring of critically ill patients. *Veterinary Technician the Complete Journal for the Veterinary Hospital Staff* **25**(7): 468-480.

L. Waddell (2008) Monitoring the cardiovascular compromised patient. International Veterinary Emergency and Critical Care Symposium.

Chapter 4
Nutritional Notability

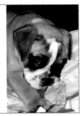

Nutritional considerations of veterinary patients can largely influence healing and recovery. Patients should be assessed individually and a nutritional plan instituted based on the underlying disease and specific needs of the patient. In essence, nutrition should be applied as an addition to medical therapeutics, helping to harmonize the dynamics of veterinary care.

There are six fundamental nutrients animals need: protein, carbohydrates, fats, vitamins, minerals, and water. These nutrients can be divided into energy-producing and non-energy-producing nutrients. Energy-producing nutrients produce energy through the processes of digestion, metabolism, and conversion. Non-energy-producing nutrients are essential for certain metabolic processes to take place.

Energy-producing nutrients: Proteins, carbohydrates, and fats

Proteins are made up of amino acids. There are essential amino acids which are required in a diet, and nonessential amino acids which the body can synthesize if needed. Protein is used for building muscle, organs, and other body tissues as well as playing a role in hormonal processes and enzymes. Once protein has been used for these purposes, it will then be used for energy, albeit less efficient energy when compared to the energy from carbohydrates and fats.

Carbohydrates have the primary function of providing energy and are classified as either soluble or insoluble. Soluble carbohydrates can be used for energy immediately by the body, whereas insoluble carbohydrates are not digestible, but can be beneficial in regulating intestinal peristalsis, blood glucose levels, and aid in weight loss. Unused carbohydrates are stored by the body, either in the liver as glycogen or as fat.

Clinical Small Animal Care: Promoting Patient Health through Preventative Nursing, First Edition.
Kimm Wuestenberg.
© 2012 John Wiley & Sons, Inc. Published 2012 by John Wiley & Sons, Inc.

Fats contain more concentrated energy than any other nutrient and are made up of essential fatty acids. Essential fatty acids influence metabolism, skin and hair health, and hormone synthesis as well as other body processes. Fats are beneficial in improving the palatability of foods and increasing the caloric density. The more fat a diet contains, the higher the calories it contains.

Non-energy-producing nutrients: Vitamins, minerals, and water

Vitamins are only required in small amounts, yet they play a large role in maintaining physiological functions. Vitamins are either water soluble or fat soluble. Water-soluble vitamins are absorbed by the small intestines. The body does not store excess water-soluble vitamins and the remainders are excreted in urine. Fat-soluble vitamins, however, are stored by the body in the liver or in fat.

Minerals, which can be divided into macrominerals or microminerals, are necessary to ensure normal metabolic processes take place. Macrominerals play a role in processes such as electrolyte and water balance, acid–base balance, muscle contraction, and nerve conduction. Microminerals, or "trace" minerals, are utilized for biochemical processes in the body. Minerals work closely together and when there is an overabundance of one mineral, another may then become deficient.

Water is the most essential nutrient required, providing the basis for metabolism of all other nutrients. In adults, 70% of body weight is made up of water. Water deficiency can lead to devastating effects such as an inability to absorb vitamins or excrete waste via the renal system, resulting in serious illness and even death (Table 4.1).

Nutritional differences between dogs and cats

There are differences in physiological nutritional needs and the institution of nutritional delivery between dogs and cats. Dogs are more likely to eat while hospitalized and if not eating on their own, can be coaxed or syringe fed with less difficulty than cats. Patients refusing to eat should be assessed for pain or inability to eat on their own, such as patients suffering from vestibular disease. Many techniques can be used to encourage eating. Hand feeding is very rewarding to both the patient and the caregiver and helps establish a bond.

A small amount of food may be placed on the patients' nose or front paw, so that the food can be tasted when the patient licks the area. Once the patient tastes the food, they are often eager to continue eating. This is especially the case in patients suffering from decreased olfactory senses, such as upper respiratory infections. Warming the meals can also help strengthen the odor and promote eating.

Some patients prefer particular feeding dishes, ranging from ceramic bowls to paper plates. Occasionally, attempting to feed a reluctant patient with a spoon may be a successful method if the owner has a tendency to share their meals with their pet. Additionally, some pets prefer dry to canned food or vice versa. If a patient is continuously reluctant to eat, the pet owner should be asked about the normal diet eaten. A

Table 4.1 Nutritional formula guideline

Steps	Formula
START with resting energy requirements (RER)	$30 \times kg + 70 = $ BASIC 24-hour caloric requirements
Then ADD individual factors:	
Canine maintenance energy requirements (MER)	
Growth < 4 months	RER × 3
Growth > 4 months	RER × 2
Adult	RER × 1.6
Geriatric	RER × 1.4
Gestation	RER × 1.8 (early) to 3 (late)
Lactation	RER × 4–8 (or ad lib)
Working	RER × 2–8 (light to heavy work load, respectively)
Feline maintenance energy requirements (MER)	
Growth	RER × 2.5
Adult	RER × 1.2
Geriatric	RER × 1.1
Gestation	RER × 1.6 (early) to 2.0 (late)
Lactation	Ad lib
Multiply by illness factors	
Cage rest	MER × 1.0–1.2
Postoperative	MER × 1.2–1.5
Trauma or sepsis	MER × 1.2–1.5

least desirable diet for the patient is better than no nutrition at all. This is especially the case in cats as they are at risk of developing hepatic lipidosis with an episode of anorexia.

If hand feeding, spoon feeding, and coaxing are not successful, the patient should be syringe fed so long as it does not cause harm (anxiety, stress) to the patient and the digestive tract is functional. There are instances where delivering nutrition parenterally or with the use of enteral tubes is required to meet nutritional requirements safely. Ill or injured patients require higher calories to sustain an increase in metabolic rate or catabolism will ensue. When nutrition is inadequate, the patient is at risk for a longer hospital stay, delayed wound healing, immunosuppression, muscle weakness, low serum albumin levels, and, in cases where bacterial translocation occurs, sepsis, organ failure and death (Figs. 4.1 and 4.2, Tables 4.2 and 4.3).

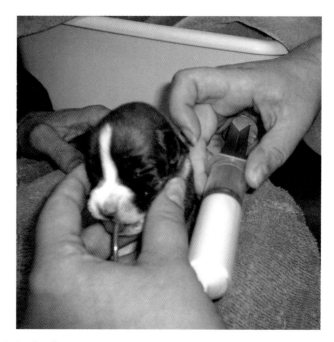

Figure 4.1 Tube feeding a neonate.

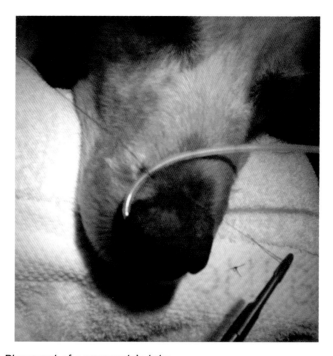

Figure 4.2 Placement of a nasogastric tube.

Table 4.2 Nursing implications

Disease state considerations	Dietary modifications	Clinical applications
Congestive heart failure	Fish oil supplement	Reduce inflammatory cytokines, decrease cachexia, may improve food intake
	Sodium restriction	May allow lower dosages of diuretics
	High quality protein	Helps meet maintenance requirements (unless kidney disease is present) and maintain lean body mass
	Potassium assessment	Loop diuretics can contribute to hypokalemia while potassium-sparing diuretics can contribute to hyperkalemia
	Taurine supplement	Supplement in diet-related dilated cardiomyopathy (DCM) in cats or metabolic defects in dogs. May have positive inotropic effects and help regulate calcium in myocardium
	n-3 fatty acids supplement	Reduce inflammation, suppress arrhythmias, improve appetite (avoid flaxseed oil and cod liver oil)
Chronic renal failure	Protein restrictions	In advanced renal failure, uremia
	Phosphorus restriction	Slows progression of renal disease
	Avoid acidifying diets	Can contribute to metabolic acidosis
Diabetes mellitus	Fiber	Calorie dense, reducing weight and insulin requirements, may help glucose regulation (primarily beneficial in dogs)
	High protein, low carbohydrate	In cats, can help reduce insulin requirements or eliminate need for insulin in some cases
Urolithiasis	Canned diet	Decrease urine specific gravity, particularly in cats
	Acidifying diet	Reduce recurrence of struvite and calcium oxalate stones, may not be necessary in dogs with struvites
	Evaluate supplements	Vitamin C will acidify urine, vitamin D can contribute to hypercalciuria

Table 4.3 Nutrient summary

Energy producing	Proteins
	Carbohydrates
	Fats
Non-energy producing	Vitamins
	Minerals
	Water

Chapter references and further reading

L. Freeman (2008a) Take-out nutrition: what to send the sick ones home with. International Veterinary Emergency and Critical Care Symposium.

L. Freeman (2008b) Nutrition in the critically ill: then and now. International Veterinary Emergency and Critical Care Symposium.

J. Hurst (2004) Feeding dogs and cats: different needs for different stages. *Veterinary Technician the Complete Journal for the Veterinary Hospital Staff* **25**(8): 538-547.

D. Proulx (2003a) Critical care nutrition I. Western Veterinary Conference.

D. Proulx (2003b) Critical care nutrition II. Western Veterinary Conference.

M. Scherk (2009) Feline nutrition. *The National Association of Veterinary Technicians in America Journal* **Winter**: 38-44.

J. Womack (2003) Providing nutritional support to critical care patients. *Veterinary Technician the Complete Journal for the Veterinary Hospital Staff* **24**(6): 376-386.

A. Wortinger (2002) Refeeding syndrome: too much of a good thing. *Veterinary Technician the Complete Journal for the Veterinary Hospital Staff* **23**(12): 724-728.

A. Wortinger (2004) Feeding habits of cats. *Veterinary Technician the Complete Journal for the Veterinary Hospital Staff* **25**(11): 762-765.

A. Wortinger (2009) The benefits of using nutrition in the management of critical care cases. *Veterinary Technician the Complete Journal for the Veterinary Hospital Staff* **30**(3): 26-28.

D. Zoran (2003) Critical care nutrition. Western Veterinary Conference.

Section 2
Applied Nursing of the Veterinary Patient

Chapter 5
Monitoring the Fluid Therapy Patient

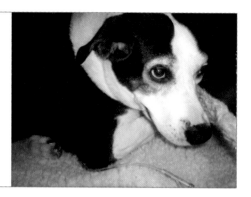

Fluid therapy is used to treat conditions such as dehydration and shock, to correct electrolyte abnormalities, and to maintain homeostasis during anesthetic and surgical procedures. The administration of fluid therapy is an important, everyday task in the veterinary profession that requires knowledge and understanding of mathematical formulas, routes of delivery, fluid selections, common additives used, and potential risks involved. It is important to recognize that not all veterinary fluid therapy cases are treated with a standard formula. Many times medical conditions such as cardiac, pulmonary, or even cerebral disorders may require an alteration of the fluid therapy plan for the patients' safety.

Mechanisms of fluid therapy

The body is comprised of 60% water in healthy adult animals and 80% water in neonates. Two-thirds of that volume is intracellular, mostly found in skeletal muscles, blood cells, bone cells, and adipose tissue. The remaining one-third resides in extracellular spaces such as blood vessels and tissues. Furthermore, one-quarter of that volume is intravascular in the form of plasma and three-quarters remain in interstitial spaces. Fluid within cells is termed intracellular fluid (ICF), and fluid outside the cells (vessels and tissue) is termed extracellular fluid (ECF).

Fluid movement occurs through capillaries, which have selectively permeable membranes. Water moves from less concentrated solutions to more concentrated solutions through this membrane (osmosis). Osmotic pressure is the force that moves fluid to create an equal balance between ICFs and ECFs. Osmotic pressure is exerted by the number of particles present (plasma osmolality), not the mass (weight) of the particles. "Tonicity" is a common term used when referring to osmotic pressure.

Electrolytes also play a major role in fluid movement because electrolytes are dissolved mainly in water. Electrolytes are considered balanced when their concentration

Clinical Small Animal Care: Promoting Patient Health through Preventative Nursing, First Edition. Kimm Wuestenberg.
© 2012 John Wiley & Sons, Inc. Published 2012 by John Wiley & Sons, Inc.

in fluid compartments remains normal and constant. Balance is primarily obtained through reabsorption of sodium and potassium.

Fluid selections for the veterinary patient

There are two main types of fluids used in veterinary medicine, crystalloids and colloids. Crystalloids are isotonic solutions that do not have osmotic pressure; therefore, they are freely passed from the intravascular space to the interstitial space. Crystalloids contain electrolytes and when they are administered intravenously, within 1 hour 20% of those fluids will remain in circulation while 80% moves into interstitial spaces to rehydrate tissues. Colloids (albumin, globulin, and fibrinogen) remain intravascular for a longer period of time because they have a large molecular weight and surface area; therefore, they cannot easily pass through the small openings in the selectively permeable membranes.

Table 5.1 lists the commonly used fluids in the veterinary practice and their purpose.

Fluid administration routes

Fluids can be administered in a variety of routes (Fig. 5.1). The most common routes include oral, subcutaneous, and intravenous. Other routes that can be used, but less frequently, include intraperitoneal and intraosseous.

Subcutaneous fluids are generally used in mild cases of dehydration and are a great choice when hospitalization isn't required but fluid therapy is still indicated. Subcutaneous fluids should not be used in severely dehydrated or debilitated patients. Fluid of choice would be an isotonic, nonirritating fluid (dextrose should not be given subcutaneously [SQ]) and no more than 10 mL/lb. given at each injection site to ensure complications (such as sloughing) do not arise.

The intravenous route of administration is the preferred method for severely ill or injured patients. Intravenous fluid therapy is more invasive than oral and subcutaneous routes as it does require the use of a catheter. However, it is a more rapid route and volumes can be given at a controlled, precise rate (Fig. 5.2).

Fluid therapy calculations

There are three fundamental goals in fluid therapy: Replace the existing fluid loss (deficit), prevent further loss (maintenance), and replace further losses (contemporary or ongoing losses).

Deficit volume

The deficit volume is the amount of fluids the patient has lost prior to clinical presentation. Some causes for fluid loss include, but are not limited to, vomit, diarrhea, anorexia, hemorrhage, and heat exhaustion.

There are three main pieces of information we can use to determine a deficit volume: The physical findings, the packed cell volume (PCV), and the estimated fluid loss. Since

Table 5.1 Common fluid selection

Crystalloids	Tonicity	Uses
0.9% NaCl (physiological saline)	Isotonic	Hyponatremia, hyperkalemia, hypercalcemia, metabolic alkalosis, renal failure, diabetes mellitus
0.45% saline with 2.5% dextrose	Hypotonic (mildly)	Heart disease (congestive heart failure [CHF]), liver disease, edema, ascites
Dextrose 5% in water	Hypotonic	Hypernatremia, sodium-intolerant patients, sepsis, provide intracellular carbohydrate source, provides free water (should not be given SQ)
LRS	Isotonic	Shock, maintenance, deficit replacement, diuresis, acidosis (has calcium)
Normosol	Isotonic	Shock, maintenance, deficit replacement, diuresis, acidosis (does not have calcium)
3% normal saline	Hypertonic	Rapidly increase intravascular volume (shock, trauma, gastric dilatation-volvulus [GDV])
Colloids	**Contents**	**Uses**
Whole blood	All cellular and plasma components	Anemia, blood loss
Plasma (FFP, platelet-enriched plasma [PEP])	Natural colloids (albumin and globulin)	Hypoproteinemia, liver disease, and volume replacement
Hemoglobin-based oxygen carriers	Hemoglobin-based, oxygen-carrying fluid	Anemia
Hetastarch	Synthetic colloid (hydroxyethyl starch and saline)	Hypovolemic shock, hypoproteinemia

the owner is usually the estimator of fluid loss prior to arrival, this method is usually the least reliable method of determining a deficit volume (see Appendix 1).

Physical findings

In order to determine a deficit volume by the patient's physical findings, this simple formula can be used (Table 5.2):

$$\text{Deficit volume (mL)} = \%\text{ dehydrated} \times \text{body weight (lb.)} \times 454 \times 0.80.$$

The percent dehydrated is based on an examination. The number 0.80 is used because only 80% of the fluid deficit should be replaced. Administering the full deficit while adding the maintenance requirements may increase the risk of fluid overload.

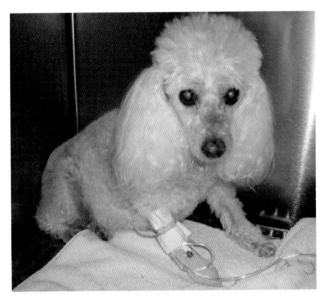

Figure 5.1 Patient receiving intravenous fluid therapy with protective catheter care instituted.

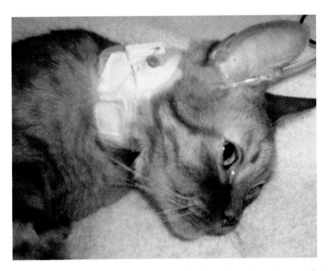

Figure 5.2 Central venous catheter placed in the jugular vein when peripheral access could not be obtained.

PCV method

Another method for determining the fluid deficit is by using a simple blood test, the PCV. For every percent increase in the PCV, there is a 10 mL/kg deficit. The normal PCV in dogs is 45% and in cats is 35%. The formula is written as follows:

$$\text{Deficit replacement volume} = 10\ \text{mL} \times \text{kg} \times \%\ \text{in PCV increase.}$$

Table 5.2   Clinical determination of dehydration severity

Percent dehydrated	Physical attributes
<5%	History of fluid loss, but no physical findings
5%	Dry mucous membrane (MM) (tacky), but no panting or pathological tachycardia
7%	Mild to moderate decrease in skin turgor, dry MM, slightly tachycardic, normal pulse pressure
10%	Moderate to marked decrease in skin turgor, dry MM, tachycardic, decreased pulse pressure
12%	Marked loss of skin turgor, dry MM, significant signs of shock

Estimated losses

This is the least reliable method as owners are generally unable to accurately determine fluid quantities since fluids tend to absorb into blankets, towels, carpets, or spread over a hard surface such as tile. As a general rule, it is assumed that animals with vomiting and diarrhea lose 4 mL/kg/day.

Maintenance volume

Calculating the maintenance volume is the next step in determining the fluid therapy regimen. Maintenance volume is the normal amount of fluid that an animal should consume to maintain homeostasis; consider it their "eight glasses of water a day."

The following is the formula for maintenance volume calculation:

$$\text{24-hour maintenance volume (mL)} = 30 \times \text{kg} + 70.$$

The total fluid volume can then be further divided to gather an hourly rate. After the 24-hour period, another exam or PCV should be performed to reevaluate the hydration status and then once again obtain a fluid regimen for the next 24 hours. Patients receiving fluids should always receive close monitoring, with appropriate modifications based on frequent reassessments.

Contemporary losses

Contemporary or ongoing losses are fluid losses that occur after a fluid therapy regimen has begun. It is assumed that fluid losses are often underestimated when visually inspected. As a common guideline, the ongoing losses are calculated by doubling the volume lost. The rate of replacing ongoing losses will depend on the amount of fluid lost and the size and overall health of the patient.

$$\text{Ongoing losses} = 2 \times \text{volume lost.}$$

Fluid additives

It is often necessary to supplement patient fluids with certain nutrients. For instance, an animal that has been vomiting or has diarrhea may have a low potassium level or a neonatal patient may have trouble regulating glucose levels and may need dextrose supplementation.

It is important to take into consideration appropriate calculations when fluids require additives. Miscalculating potassium may have lethal effects as hyperkalemia (high potassium blood levels) may result in cardiac failure. Potassium is supplied in mEq/mL, or milliequivalents per milliliter, as opposed to the more commonly seen unit of measurement, milligrams. Milliequivalents are a unit of measurement used for electrolytes because it is expressing the number of ionic charges.

To calculate mEq additives you can use this simple formula:

Desired amount (mEq)/available (stock) concentration (mEq/mL)
= amount (mL) to add.

When potassium chloride is added to fluids, it must always be mixed well by inverting the bag several times. If it is not mixed well, an overabundance of potassium may enter the administration set at a fatal concentration.

Additionally, if the total desired amount of potassium is 20 mEq/L, be aware of already existing potassium in certain fluid selections. For example, lactated Ringer's solution (LRS) contains 4 mEq/L of potassium.

The most notable fluid additive miscalculations occur when a percent solution is required, such as 50% dextrose. A percent (%) is a concentration unit per 100 in which the item of importance precedes the percent symbol. Two components make up a percent solution, the solute (item) and the solvent (the item in which the solute is dissolved).

A simple formula to calculate percentage solutions is as follows:

$$\frac{\text{Desired strength of solution}}{\text{Available strength in stock}} = \frac{\text{Volume of stock solution to use}}{\text{Total volume of solution}}.$$

Example:

$$\frac{2.5\%}{50\%} = \frac{X\,mL}{100\,mL}.$$

Two and a half percent (2.5%) is the desired concentration; X is the unknown amount to use; 50% is the available drug strength; and 100 is the total amount to make.

Cross-multiply and divide:

$$\frac{2.5}{50} \times \frac{X}{100} = \frac{250}{50X} \quad X = 5\,mL.$$

Adding 5 mL of a 50% solute will create a 2.5% solution. However, by adding 5 mL of solute to 100 mL of solvent, there is now a total of 105 mL, as opposed to the 100 mL desired. Thus, 5 mL of the solvent must be removed prior to adding 5 mL of the solute

Table 5.3 Common fluid additives

Common fluid additives	Use
Potassium chloride (KCl)	Vomiting, diuresis, hypokalemia
Dextrose (2.5%, 5%, etc.)	Hypoglycemia, anorexia, sepsis, hyperthyroidism
Vitamin B complex	Anorexia

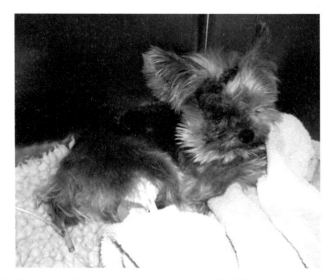

Figure 5.3 Patient receiving long-term intravenous fluid therapy post-rattlesnake envenomation.

to keep an accurate 2.5% solution. When performing calculations, it is imperative to arrange the numbers in proper units of measurement. For example, if the above problem required a total amount of 1 L, it would need to be converted to 1000 mL prior to calculating (Table 5.3).

Monitoring the patient

All animals receiving fluid therapy should be carefully monitored (Fig. 5.3). Too little fluid can lead to dehydration and hypotension and an overdose of fluids can lead to pulmonary edema and even death. As the fluid therapy patient stabilizes, adjustments to the rate of fluid administration and type of fluids required may be necessary. These adjustments can be made by performing laboratory tests such as packed cell volume and total solids (PCV/TS) and electrolytes and also by observing clinical changes with the patient such as vomiting, indicating fluids are needed, or excessive urination, which may indicate the patient is well hydrated.

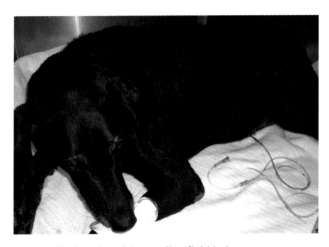

Figure 5.4 Urinary catheter placed to monitor fluid balances.

Unfortunately, a common problem that occurs while administering fluid therapy is running off-schedule with the delivery rate and time. This may be due to the patient resting in a way that occludes the flow, or conversely, standing and allowing a rush of fluids to enter the vein. In either case, the fluid rate needs to be recalculated but the emphasis on critical thinking comes in to play when the fluids are running behind schedule to avoid fluid overload.

Signs and symptoms of fluid overload include nasal secretions (usually a clear nasal discharge), tachycardia, lung sounds upon auscultation, coughing, and restlessness. Patients receiving fluid therapy should routinely have their lungs auscultated. In the early stages of fluid overload, the patient may exhibit trembling, nausea or vomiting, and possibly excitation, panting, or tachypnea. Another key indicator is polyuria. Normal urine output is 1-2 mL/kg/h. If these subtle symptoms are missed by the caregiver, then serious fluid overloading can ensue. Clinical signs of serious overloading include tachycardia, bradycardia in severe late cases, nasal discharge, cough, dyspnea, subcutaneous edema, chemosis, or exophthalmia. Patients may also suffer from diarrhea, depression, pulmonary edema, and pleural effusion (Fig. 5.4).

Fluid balances should be assessed at least once daily in the stable patient, and more frequently in debilitated patients, particularly those suffering from renal disease or hypotension. Urine production generally reflects overall tissue perfusion. With each cardiac cycle, the kidneys receive 25% of cardiac output. Normal urine output is 1-2 mL/kg/h; by quantitating urine output, a rough assessment of tissue perfusion can be obtained. Additionally, other excretory means such as diarrhea, emesis, or even pleural fluid from a chest tube should be calculated in the fluid balancing. Patients should be weighed at least once a day, with critical patients at risk of third spacing fluid shifts being weighed up to every 2-4 hours as part of the balancing. Fluid balancing is imperative in recognizing underhydration, overhydration, and organ function (Table 5.4, Figs. 5.5-5.7).

Table 5.4 Fluid therapy nursing implications

Fluid therapy nursing implications	Frequency	Reasoning
Patient weight	At least once a day, more frequently for renal or hypoproteinemic patients	Body weight changes can indicate diuresis or fluid retention, can detect third spacing of fluids
Physical assessment	Every 2–6 hours, depending on clinical condition	Evaluate hydration, prevent dehydration or overhydration, monitor patient fluid delivery route for extravasation, assess patient needs
Fluid balances	Every 4–12 hours based on clinical condition	Early recognition of oliguria, prevent anuria; early recognition of fluid overload
Laboratory testing	Every 24 hours, or as needed if warranted	Monitor hydration status, detect iatrogenic anemia (hemodilution), detect electrolyte abnormalities

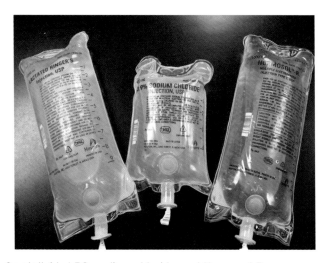

Figure 5.5   Crystalloids LRS, sodium chloride, and Normosol-R.

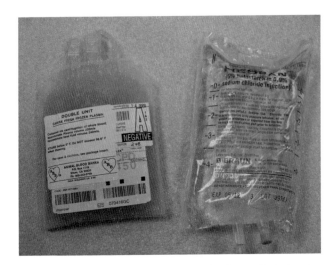

Figure 5.6 Colloids fresh frozen plasma (FFP) and hydroxyethyl starch.

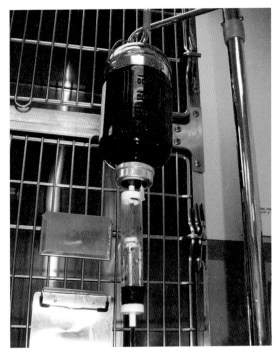

Figure 5.7 Whole blood.

Chapter references and further reading

T. Hackett (2008) Fluid therapy. *The National Association of Veterinary Technicians in America Journal* **Summer**: 58–63.

P. Hellyer (2002) Fluid therapy: a cornerstone of safe anesthesia. *The National Association of Veterinary Technicians in America Journal* **Winter**: 35–38.

J. Kerr (2009) Fluid therapy: a team approach to patient hydration. *Veterinary Technician the Complete Journal for the Veterinary Hospital Staff* **30**(5): 16–23.

B. Rieser (2003) Logical fluid therapy. Western Veterinary Conference.

Chapter 6
Physical Therapy Applications

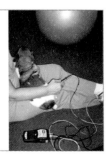

Physical therapy, often referred to as physiotherapy, is defined as the science of applying biomechanics, physics, anatomy, physiology, and psychology to individuals with dysfunction, injury, or pain. Physical therapy enhances the natural healing process and improves surgery or injury recovery time. Physical therapy also increases blood flow, allows for better lymph drainage, prevents or reduces muscle atrophy, and reduces pain. In the recumbent patient, thoracic physical therapy helps improve breathing, thus increasing oxygen in systemic circulation. In addition, physical therapy is a noninvasive treatment, is generally low cost, and has psychological benefits for the patient. The main forethought in performing physical therapy is having an accurate understanding of the nature of the injury and the mechanism(s) involved in recovery. The use of physical therapy in the critical patient can help prevent secondary conditions from arising. Critical or recumbent patients often suffer from secondary illnesses such as atelectasis, pneumonia, thrombosis, and muscle atrophy. Instituting a physical therapy plan in the intensive care unit (ICU) has many benefits for the patient.

Techniques which are useful to the ICU patient include massage, active and passive range of motion (ROM, PROM), thermal agents, positioning, postural drainage, percussion, vibration, and low level lasers. Physical therapy can be performed every 4–8 hours depending on the patients' needs. Massage and ROM exercises will help circulation, reducing the risk for thrombosis. ROM exercises will help prevent or reduce muscle atrophy. Thermal agents include the application of heat and/or ice. While heat dilates the capillaries and allows for better blood flow to the region, ice will cause vasoconstriction, reducing swelling and inflammation. Furthermore, both of these thermal agents contribute to pain management. Positional changes help prevent decubitus ulcers, atelectasis, and peripheral edema. Postural drainage, percussion, and vibration should be implemented in the ICU patient due to the inability to productively cough. Activity stimulates coughing; therefore, the recumbent, obtunded, or comatose patient may accumulate respiratory secretions and suffer from conditions such as pneumonia as a sequela (Figs. 6.1 and 6.2).

Clinical Small Animal Care: Promoting Patient Health through Preventative Nursing, First Edition.
Kimm Wuestenberg.

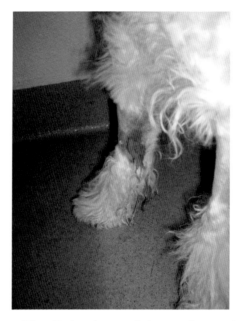

Figure 6.1 Intravenous (IV) catheter abscess 4 days postremoval.

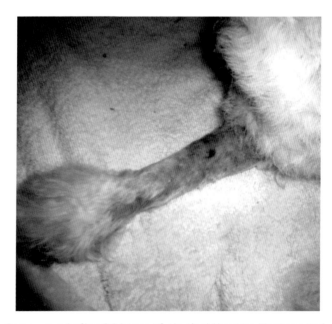

Figure 6.2 Same wound after 24 hours of physical therapy. Massage and hydrotherapy was used.

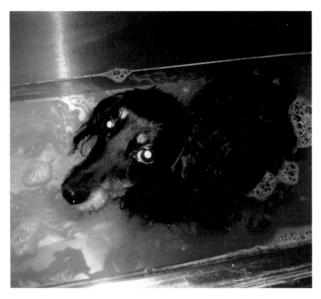

Figure 6.3 Swim therapy in a dachshund with intervertebral disk disease (IVDD) suffering hind limb paresis following thromboembolism.

Massage therapy relaxes the patient and aids in pain relief. There are two main massage techniques used in a critical care setting—effleurage and petrissage. Petrissage involves a squeezing and kneading technique while effleurage involves strokes. Both techniques improve circulation, and thus should be performed distal to proximal on the extremities.

Rehabilitation exercises such as ROM and PROM are used in the ICU to improve circulation and prevent peripheral edema in addition to preventing muscle atrophy. The extremities should be flexed and extended prior to ROM exercises. In PROM, the veterinary personnel are moving the extremities and the joints in a slow cycling motion, while active ROM involves the patient actively moving and resisting. Several sets are performed two to three times daily, with care being taken to not overexert the patient (Fig. 6.3).

Thermal agents, as mentioned above, will provide analgesia and reduce inflammation. The application of cold packs is typically used within the first 24-48 hours of injury or surgery every 4-6 hours. After the initial 24 to 48-hour period, heat is then used at the same interval schedule. Care should be taken to prevent patient burns. A towel should be placed between the agent and the patient when heat and cold applications are used. Thermal agents can be applied for 5-15 minutes at each session (Fig. 6.4).

Positional changes involve moving a patient from right lateral, to sternal, to left lateral recumbency throughout the hospital stay. Decubital ulcers, pneumonia, and atelectasis may ensue if the patient is not moved for a significant period of time. Adequate blankets, pillows, cushions, and mattresses should be used in the recumbent patient to aid in positioning and preventing pressure sores (Table 6.1).

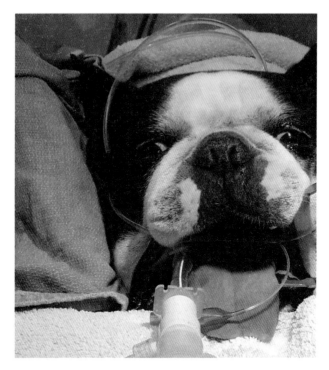

Figure 6.4 Application of a thermal agent, in this case an ice pack, in a Boston terrier with severe edema.

Thoracic physical therapy, or chest physiotherapy (CPT), includes postural drainage, percussion, and vibration. Other treatments that may be used in conjunction with thoracic physical therapy include nebulization and suctioning of secretions. Percussion, or coupage, is performed by cupping the hands and gently impacting the thorax during inhalation and exhalation. This technique helps break up secretions. Vibration can then be performed to help further break up secretions and move them toward the larger airways. Vibration is performed on exhalation and involves rapidly moving hands in a tapping motion over specific areas of the chest. Vibration is less forceful than percussion and may be used in place of percussion in patients with rib injuries. Postural drainage uses gravity to drain secretions in the lungs and into the main airway and also relieves pressure in cases of atelectasis. These secretions can either be suctioned out or, if able, the patient may cough the secretions out of the airway. Assisted cough may be required if the patient is unable to remove mucus from the airway. Assisted cough should be performed with the patient in sternal recumbency and can be induced by gently palpating the trachea. A maneuver (similar to the Heimlich maneuver) where pressure is placed on the cranial abdomen, thrusting cranially on exhalation, may also aid in coughing up secretions (Table 6.2).

Postural drainage is not without risks. There can be significant side effects such as oxygen deficiency, an increased intracranial pressure, decreased blood pressure, bleeding into the lungs, pain, vomiting (with or without aspiration), and injury to the spinal

Table 6.1 Example of potential physiotherapy interventions

ICU-specific conditions	Physical therapy techniques
Neurological (i.e., spinal cord injury, paralysis, paresis)	Positioning, PROM, massage, postural drainage with or without percussion, and vibration
Soft tissue (i.e., muscle atrophy, wound care, edema, inflammation)	Positioning, laser, PROM, massage, ice
Respiratory (i.e., pneumonia, atelectasis, mechanical ventilation)	PROM, massage, percussion, vibration, postural drainage

Table 6.2 Postural drainage techniques

Position	Action focal point
Left lateral recumbency with hind end elevated 40°	Lateral segment of left caudal lung lobe; lateral segment of the right caudal lung lobe
Sternal recumbency with hind end elevated 40°	Left and right caudal dorsal lung fields
Dorsal recumbency with hind end elevated 40°	Left and right caudal ventral lung fields
Dorsal recumbency with hind end elevated 40°, front end rotated 1/4 turn to the right with a pillow under the right side of thorax	Right middle lung lobe
Sternal recumbency with front end elevated 40°	Left and right cranial dorsal lung fields
Dorsal recumbency with front end elevated 40°	Left and right cranial ventral lung fields

cord. In human studies, cardiac arrhythmias have been noted during postural drainage and percussion of ICU patients. Human precaution guidelines to heed include patients with neck or head injuries, active hemorrhage or bleeding from the lungs, fractured ribs, recent surgeries, open wounds, burns, and pulmonary embolism. Veterinary precautions published include coagulopathies and cardiac disease in addition to the aforementioned conditions. During postural drainage, patients are placed in specific positions for up to 15 minutes, with recumbent patients receiving drainage therapy every 6–8 hours. The goal of thoracic physical therapy is to ensure the patient is able to breathe in adequate amounts of oxygen and sputum secretions are being removed from the lungs. Arterial blood gases may be performed to monitor the results of thoracic physical therapy as well as manual auscultation and assessment of lung sound changes.

Chapter references and further reading

T. McLaughlin (2009) Hydrotherapy–offering a new lease on life. *Veterinary Technician the Complete Journal for the Veterinary Hospital Staff* **30**(1): 20-23.

J. Osborne, N. Sharp (1998) Putting "wobblers" back on track. *Veterinary Technician the Complete Journal for the Veterinary Hospital Staff* **19**(8): 519-527.

V. Rhodes (2005) Osteoarthritis in a senior pet. *Veterinary Technician the Complete Journal for the Veterinary Hospital Staff* **26**(10): 702-704.

Chapter 7
Perioperative Patient Management

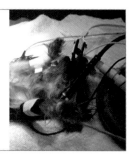

Perioperative nursing

Perioperative nursing refers to patient nursing from the preoperative time, throughout the surgical or anesthetic procedure, and care for the patient postoperatively. Surgical and anesthetic procedures are typically an everyday event in most veterinary practices. Whenever possible, it is recommended that the same veterinary technician care for the patient from the preoperative phase to the intraoperative phase and throughout the postoperative phase. This enables the nursing staff to recognize the patients' needs, vital sign trends, and any astute detection of changes in clinical conditions. Patients undergoing surgical procedure are at risk for developing nosocomial infections, therefore proper perioperative nursing is imperative to help reduce the risks of infection.

Preoperative patient nursing

Any patient undergoing an anesthetic or surgical procedure should have a physical exam performed within a reasonable amount of time prior to the procedure (such as 2-6 hours). The patient identity, procedure, and special implications, such as heart disease or adverse reactions to medication, should be confirmed. Vital signs should be assessed and documented to establish a baseline of normal values for the patient. Vital sign parameters will often alter throughout and after anesthetic procedures. Identifying normal values in each patient will help the nursing staff detect abnormalities beyond surgical and anesthetic influences.

Once the patient status and procedure has been verified and the patient has been cleared for surgery, preparation should begin. Anesthetic protocols should be established for the patient, fluid therapy calculated, and the surgical site prepared if an incision is to be made during the procedure. In an ideal situation, patients would be

Clinical Small Animal Care: Promoting Patient Health through Preventative Nursing, First Edition.
Kimm Wuestenberg.
© 2012 John Wiley & Sons, Inc. Published 2012 by John Wiley & Sons, Inc.

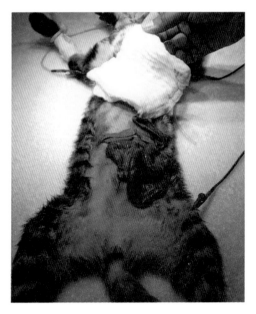

Figure 7.1 Surgical preparation of a patient with spay dehiscence.

bathed prior to surgery, removing excess debris; however, this practice is often only reserved for major surgical procedures such as total hip replacements. Care should be taken to prevent skin irritation or superficial lacerations when clipping the surgical site. Surgical site infections most commonly develop from normal skin flora, such as *Staphylococcus* and *Streptococcus*. The hair should be clipped liberally with a general guideline of the shaved region extending 20 cm from the incision. The removed hair should be vacuumed and the surgical site scrubbed with a germicidal soap. These preparations should be performed outside of the surgical suite. Once the patient has been transported to the surgical suite, a final surgical scrub (usually three separate scrubs) should ensue (Fig. 7.1).

Intraoperative patient nursing

While there are several aspects to surgical nursing, patient care and monitoring will be the focus of this section. Whenever possible, the use of multiparameter monitoring systems should be implemented, but should never take the place of hands-on patient monitoring by the veterinary technician. Starting from the head, patient care should begin with lubrication of the eyes to prevent drying of the cornea and risks of subsequent ulceration. Excess secretions in the mouth should be cleared and a patent airway verified. Once the patient is positioned for the procedure, areas exposed should be assessed for the potential to apply warming devices. The patients' body temperature should be closely monitored and proactive measures taken to prevent hypothermia (Fig. 7.2).

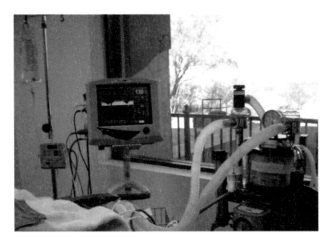

Figure 7.2 Anesthetic monitoring system.

The veterinary technician should establish at least one source to obtain a pulse throughout the procedure. Common areas include the dorsal metatarsal, femoral, jugular, and sublingual vessels. A hand may also be placed on the heart to confirm heartbeat, but monitoring pulse quality and trends or changes in the quality can be vital in detecting inadequate perfusion. Continuous monitoring of the cardiovascular system is essential during intraoperative nursing, as sudden changes can rapidly be detected, proving to be lifesaving. Electrocardiographs are useful in detecting arrhythmias commonly seen in anesthesia such as premature ventricular contractions and atrioventricular heart blocks. However, they should not be relied upon for an accurate heartbeat as electrical activity still occurs in the minutes after cardiac arrest. Blood pressure monitoring is essential because anesthesia can cause a slowed heart rate and thus lower blood pressure. The mean arterial pressure (MAP) should remain above 60 mmHg with a preferential range of 70–110 mmHg. When the MAP drops below 60 mmHg, vital organs such as the liver and kidneys are not receiving adequate perfusion, setting the patient up for serious postoperative complications like organ failure (Fig. 7.3).

Throughout the procedure, the respiratory rate and pattern should be continuously monitored in addition to repeatedly verifying the airway. Endotracheal tubes can become occluded with secretions; anesthetic tubes may become kinked or dislodged; and reservoir bags may detach, leak, or overfill. Capnographs are useful in detecting exhausted carbon dioxide absorbent, monitoring inspired and expired carbon dioxide levels, and helping in the detection of improperly placed tubes, such as placement into a mainstem bronchus.

Lastly, the depth of anesthesia and management of pain should be continuously assessed throughout the procedure. Patients can quickly become overdosed or become deficient of inhalant anesthetics. Patients should be kept in an anesthetic depth where they are not experiencing pain or sensation of surgery, but not so deep to result in dangerous vital sign parameters.

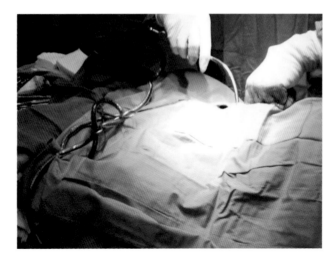

Figure 7.3 Blood pressure monitoring is especially crucial in cases of hemorrhage. This patient, Azo, suffered from a ruptured liver mass and subsequent liver lobectomy. Azo recovered well despite the hypotensive challenges experienced throughout surgery.

When the procedure is nearing the end, the patient should be reassessed and anticipation of recovery needs prepared. Some considerations include the adequate management of pain and potential for immediate postoperative pain management. The patient recovery kennel should be warmed, with sufficient clean and padded bedding for comfort. Additionally, assessment should be made for other needs such as oxygen therapy, the application of physical therapy (ice packs), or the immediate placement of an Elizabethan collar in ophthalmic surgeries.

Postoperative patient nursing

Postoperative nursing entails caring for the patient in the immediate hours following surgery and long-term monitoring when the patient remains hospitalized for days after the procedure. In initial phases of postoperative recovery, endotracheal extubation is commonly one of the first aspects. The endotracheal tube should remain inflated and intact until the patient has gained control of the gag reflex. If the endotracheal tube is removed prior to the presence of a gag reflex, the patient may be at risk for airway obstruction, such as in patients with an elongated soft palate, or aspiration pneumonia in cases of postoperative emesis. Additionally, if the cuff is deflated and the patient does not have a gag reflex, aspiration of content such as mucous secretions or even vomitus is possible. Occasionally a patient will wake violently from anesthesia, making it a difficult task to deflate the cuff and remove the tube in a timely fashion. It is imperative to prevent the patient from severing the tube by biting it or causing tracheal damage while thrashing with the tube in place. Sedatives or additional analgesics may be necessary in aiding a postsurgical or anesthetic recovery (Fig. 7.4).

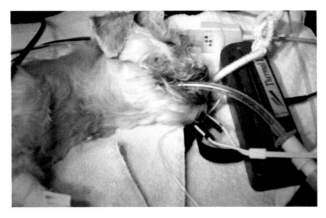

Figure 7.4 Immediate postoperative regurgitation.

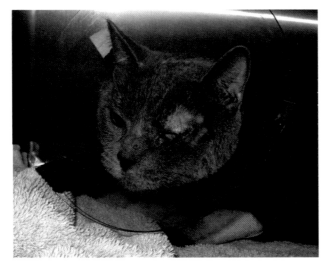

Figure 7.5 Mr. Gary Phalange recovering from phacoemulsification and lens capsulotomy for treatment of aqueous misdirection; an Elizabethan collar has been placed to prevent post-operative damage to the eye.

The patient should be monitored for heart rate, respiratory rate, and evaluated for signs of pain and level of consciousness. Once the patient is stable and alert, the intervals of assessments may increase. The surgical site should be evaluated on a regular basis for bleeding, redness, swelling, or signs of infection. Depending on the procedure performed, physical therapy interventions, serial blood tests, bandage care, continued pain management, or the administration of other medications may be warranted (Fig. 7.5, Table 7.1).

Table 7.1 Example of anesthetic monitoring flow sheet

Date:		Patient:			Owner:			Risk Factor: 1 2 3 4 5	
Procedure:						Dr:		Tech:	

PreAx Med	Strength	Dose	Route	Time	Initials	Time:	Temp:		Wt:
						HR:	RR:		MM:
						IVC			Ax Type:
						Special Concerns:			
						Fluid Type:			
						Rate:			
						Total Volume:			

Induction	Dose	Amt Given	Route	Time

Chamber	Mask	ET Tube Size:		

Monitoring:		
Pulse Ox ☐	BP	☐
ECG ☐	Temp	☐
Capnograph ☐	Other:	☐

Intra-Op	Strength	Dose	Route	Time	Initials

Ax Start:		Ax End:	
Sx Start:		Sx End:	
Extubated:			

Time:											
Ax Rate:											
O₂ Rate											
Pulse Ox:											
ETCO₂											
Temp:											
190											
180											
170											
160											
150											
140											
130											
120											
110											
100											
90											
80											
70											
60											
50											
40											
30											
20											
10											
0											

HR ●	Notes:				Post-Op	Time	HR	RR	Temp
RR ○									
Sys ⌃									
Dias ⌄									
MAP ☆									

Ax, anesthesia; PreAx Med, preanesthesia medicine; Temp, temperature; Wt, weight; HR, heart rate; RR, respiratory rate; MM, mucous membrane; IVC, intravenous catheter; Amt, amount; ET, endotracheal; Intra-Op, intraoperative; Pulse Ox, pulse oximetry; ECG, electrocardiography; Sx, surgery; BP, blood pressure; ETCO₂, end-tidal CO_2; Sys, systolic; Dias, diastolic; MAP, mean arterial pressure; Post-Op, postoperative.

Chapter references and further reading

C. Cornell (2001a) Anesthesia equipment. Wild West Veterinary Conference.

C. Cornell (2001b) High risk anesthesia. Wild West Veterinary Conference.

H. Davis (2001) Postoperative/Anesthetic nursing management of the critically ill patient. Wild West Veterinary Conference.

E. Durham (2005) Arterial blood pressure measurement. *Veterinary Technician the Complete Journal for the Veterinary Hospital Staff* **26**(5): 324-339.

S. Greene (2003) Monitoring the anesthetized patient. Western Veterinary Conference.

P. Hellyer (2002) Fluid therapy: a cornerstone of safe anesthesia. *The National Association of Veterinary Technicians in America Journal* **Winter**: 35-38.

S. Kaiser-Klinger (2008) Troubleshooting emergency anesthesia. International Veterinary Emergency and Critical Care Symposium.

V. Lukasic (2006) Anesthesia of the pediatric patient. *The National Association of Veterinary Technicians in America Journal* **Fall**: 52-57.

L. Madsen (2005) Perioperative pain management. *Veterinary Technician the Complete Journal for the Veterinary Hospital Staff* **26**(5): 359-368.

C. Mosley (2006) Anesthetic management of the geriatric patient. *The National Association of Veterinary Technicians in America Journal* **Summer**: 52-57.

B. Rhodes (2003) Hypothermia and frostbite in pets. *Veterinary Technician the Complete Journal for the Veterinary Hospital Staff* **24**(11): 750-756.

H. Ruess-Lamky (2008) Anesthetic monitors: understanding their use and limitations. *The National Association of Veterinary Technicians in America Journal* **Spring**: 60-67.

S. Shackelford (2004) Aseptic technique for surgery. *Veterinary Technician the Complete Journal for the Veterinary Hospital Staff* **25**(1): 49-52.

M. Tefend (2004) Hemodynamic monitoring of critically ill patients. *Veterinary Technician the Complete Journal for the Veterinary Hospital Staff* **25**(7): 468-480.

A. Weil (2005) Anesthetic emergencies. *The National Association of Veterinary Technicians in America Journal* **Spring**: 42-49.

Chapter 8
Executing Emergency Care

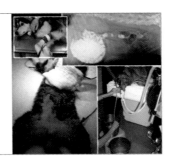

The recognition and treatment of shock continues to be a challenge in veterinary medicine. Early recognition from veterinary personnel in conjunction with prompt, efficient resuscitation efforts contribute to the successful treatment of shock. A good, general understanding of the pathophysiology of shock is not only essential in immediate resuscitation, but it is also a key indicator for anticipating events in both the prearrest and postresuscitation stages. Recognizing the clinical signs associated with shock states is imperative.

Shock is defined as a disturbance of function, an imbalance between delivered oxygen and consumed oxygen where the former is deficient. For a general background, the blood functions to deliver oxygen, nutrients, and hormones, among other necessities, to the body's tissues. The blood also carries away waste products from those tissues and it aids in the maintenance of the body's fluid balance. All tissues in the body need blood flow to deliver nutrients and carry away wastes. Oxygen delivery to the body tissues is dependent on cardiac output, which is determined by heart rate and stroke volume (consisting of cardiac preload). If cardiac function and perfusion is impaired, neurohormonal responses ensue and inflammatory mediators contribute to a vicious cycle as decompensation occurs. Oxygen has traditionally been coined "the first-line drug" in emergencies. The cardiovascular and respiratory systems should immediately be assessed and evaluated for functional oxygen delivery.

During the initial stages of shock, cellular hypoxia causes an energy deficit as mitochrondia are no longer able to generate adenosine triphosphate (ATP). Anaerobic metabolism ensues, causing the pH to fall, leading to metabolic acidosis. An acute compensatory sympathetic response causes major arteries and veins to constrict. Initially, capillaries constrict, causing a decreased perfusion to tissues; however, as anaerobic metabolism progresses, blood flow into the capillaries is increased as outflow is restricted, causing a volume shift of blood accumulating in the venules. This local "pooling" is responsible for the misdistribution of blood flow. Fluid and protein then leaks into the surrounding tissues, which concentrates the blood and increases viscosity on a microvascular level. Prolonged vasoconstriction results in loss of blood flow to

Clinical Small Animal Care: Promoting Patient Health through Preventative Nursing, First Edition. Kimm Wuestenberg.
© 2012 John Wiley & Sons, Inc. Published 2012 by John Wiley & Sons, Inc.

vital organs which were previously protected by arterial shunting. The end result is catastrophic as this terminal phase of shock is reached.

There are three defined clinical stages of shock: early (compensatory) stage, middle (decompensatory) stage, and the end (terminal) stage of shock. Vital sign parameters have been developed for each stage to better classify the progression of the shock process. When an emergent patient presents, the most life-threatening conditions should be addressed first, and quickly, to prevent further deterioration (Tables 8.1 and 8.2).

Table 8.1 Types, causes, and examples of shock

Types of shock	Cause	Examples
Hypovolemic	Low blood volume	Anemia, hemorrhage
Neurogenic	Nervous system effect	Toxins such as ethylene glycol or strychnine
Cardiogenic	Heart disease	Congestive heart failure (CHF), pericardial tamponade
Anaphylactic	Massive immune response	Bee sting, vaccination
Septic	Bacteria endotoxin	Sepsis

Table 8.2 Stages of shock

Physical parameters	Compensatory stage	Decompensatory stage	Terminal stage
Heart rate	Normal to mild elevation	Tachycardia	Severe bradycardia
Pulse quality	Normal to bounding	Poor	Absent
Blood pressure	Normal	Hypotension	Severe hypotension
Respiratory rate	Eupneic or mild elevation	Tachypnea	Bradypnea or apnea
Mucous membrane (MM)	Normal to injected	Pallor	Pallor
Capillary refill time (CRT)	<1 second	>2 seconds	>5 seconds or absent
Temperature	Euthermic or slightly elevated	Hypothermia	Profound hypothermia
Mentation	Normal, alert, or excited	Depressed or obtunded	Stuporous or comatose
Physiological effects of shock	Neurohormonal (neuroendocrine) response, hypermetabolic	Shunting of blood to vital organs, O_2 consumption dependant on O_2 delivery, metabolic acidosis	Dysfunctional blood flow, *circulus vitiosis*, impending CPA

Initial assessments of the emergent patient

A CRASH PLAN is an acronym for a guide in the assessment of body organs and systems. By utilizing this acronym, one can be sure to include every aspect of assessing the emergent patient. This assessment should be performed very quickly, in a matter of a few short minutes (Table 8.3).

Airway

Check the patient for breathing. If they are not breathing, check for an obstruction of the airway. Oftentimes there is a tennis ball or bone that has become lodged, asphyxiating (suffocating) the pet (Figs. 8.1-8.3).

Table 8.3   A CRASH PLAN

Acronym
Airway
Circulation
Respiratory
Abdomen
Spine
Head
Pelvis
Limbs
Arteries and veins
Nerves

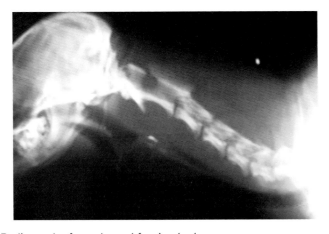

Figure 8.1   Radiograph of esophageal foreign body.

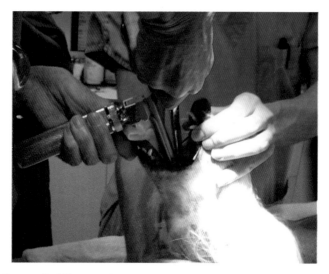

Figure 8.2 Removal of the esophageal foreign body.

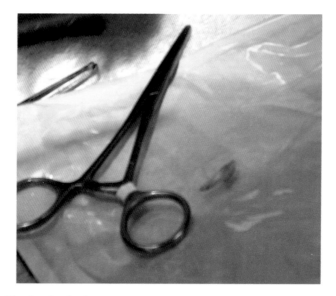

Figure 8.3 The foreign body.

Circulation

Check the patient for a heartbeat and for pulse quality. If there is no heartbeat and no pulses can be palpated, then cardiopulmonary cerebral resuscitation (CPCR) should begin at this time.

Respiratory

Observe the patient's chest. Watch for a rise and fall indicating respirations. A hand may also be placed in front of the mouth or nose to feel for a breath. If the patient is

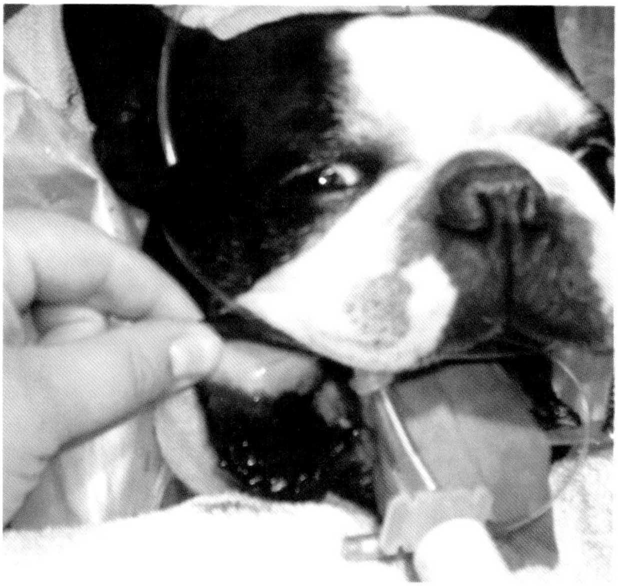

Figure 8.4 Intubation due to edema-induced asphyxiation in a rattlesnake envenomation patient.

apneic (not breathing), then manual (artificial) respirations should be performed. Mouth-to-snout resuscitation can be used until an endotracheal or transtracheal airway can be established (Fig. 8.4).

Abdomen

Take note of any swelling of the abdomen or any perforations in the abdomen. An evisceration is where the abdominal organs have herniated through the abdominal wall. This can occur with dog bite wounds, vehicle accidents, and other traumas. In this case, it is best to wrap a sterile, saline-soaked lap sponge (no cotton) over the area until surgical correction can be performed. Impalement occurs when an object has become lodged into an animal, such as trying to jump a fence or falling from heights. The important thing to remember with impalement is that the object should never be removed from the pet, as it is most likely acting as a pressure point to several arteries and vessels. Removing an impaled object can result in a lethal hemorrhage (Fig. 8.5).

Swelling should be assessed immediately to decipher between fluid and air. The veterinarian will make the diagnosis, but it is important for nursing personnel to understand the clinical presentation of each condition as either of these conditions can pose a life-threatening emergency. If the abdomen is air filled as in a GDV (gastric dilatation-volvulus), a gastrocentesis should be performed to relieve the pressure on the abdominal aorta and vena cava, improving circulation. If the abdomen is fluid filled, a diagnostic abdominocentesis should be performed. Ascites can be relieved by therapeutic abdominocentesis, where a pressure bandage may be beneficial in a hemoabdomen and surgery may be required for peritonitis (Figs. 8.6-8.8).

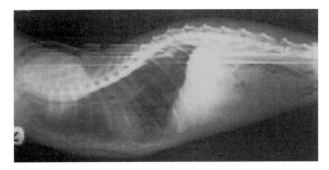

Figure 8.5 Arrow impalement of cat.

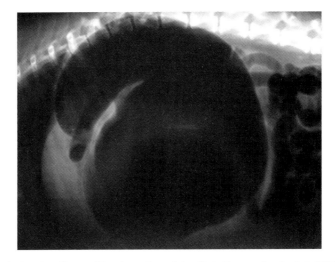

Figure 8.6 Lateral radiographic view of gastric dilatation and volvulus (GDV).

Spine

If the patient is nonambulatory, it is recommended to keep them flat in lateral recumbency until a neurological and orthopedic exam can be performed. If the pet has a history of back disease or is showing clinical signs of back problems, such as hunching the back, dragging the hind legs, or exhibiting ataxia, the patient's spine should be kept as even as possible to prevent any further damage (Fig. 8.9).

Head

Along with mentation, the head should be examined for any wounds indicating head trauma. A PLR (pupillary light reflex) can also help determine head trauma. Pupils should be equal and they should respond (constrict) when shined with a light. If head trauma is suspected, it is generally recommended to elevate the head slightly with a towel, pillow, or blanket (Figs. 8.10 and 8.11).

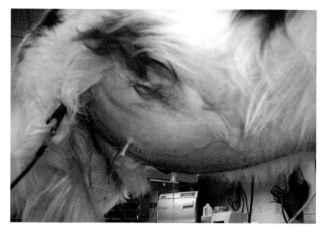

Figures 8.7 Therapeutic abdominocentesis in congestive heart failure (CHF).

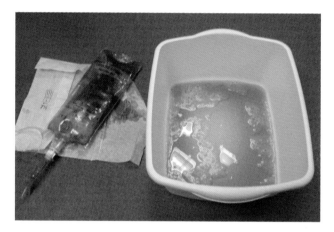

Figures 8.8 Abdominal fluid palliatively removed from a boxer with heart failure.

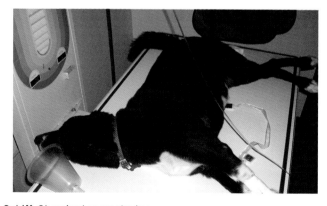

Figure 8.9 Schiff–Sherrington posturing.

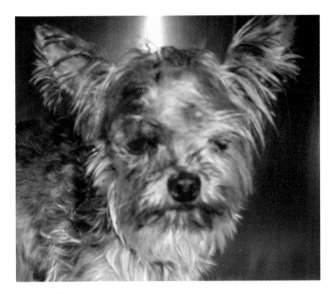

Figure 8.10 Patient with head trauma.

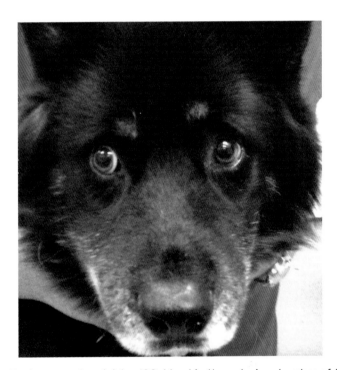

Figure 8.11 Hyphema *oculus sinister* (OS; blood in the anterior chamber of the left eye).

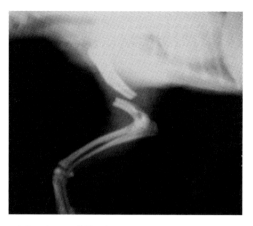

Figure 8.12 Compound fracture of the humerus.

Pelvis

A very common sequela of motor vehicle accident is a hip luxation, where the femoral head is no longer in the socket of the hip. Pelvic fractures are also common with trauma. If a pelvic fracture is noted, urine output must be monitored while the patient is in the hospital to ensure normal function of the bladder.

Limbs

Limbs should be assessed for open wounds and fractures. It is recommended to stabilize a fracture until surgical correction (or casting/splinting) can be performed. Any and all wounds should be clipped free of hair and properly disinfected to prevent a secondary bacterial infection. Bacteria grow at the rate of 10^6 every hour; the sooner the wound is cleaned, the better for the pet (Fig. 8.12).

Arteries and veins

Survey the patient for bleeding. Pressure or pressure bandages should be applied to bleeding wounds until hemostasis has been achieved. Oftentimes, an artery has been severed and surgical intervention is needed. The forceful use of a tourniquet may cause nerve or tissue damage, thus special care should be taken when applying a tourniquet to achieve hemostasis. Generally a soft bandage, placed with mild to moderate pressure, will control bleeding.

Nerves

It is important to note the patients' awareness of all body parts. Damage can occur to a nerve, nerve root, or nerve plexus due to trauma. Toxicosis may also result in nervous system dysfunction. Quick assessments that are used include proprioception and reflex tests. Proprioception is where the pet's paw is turned over so the dorsal aspect is now

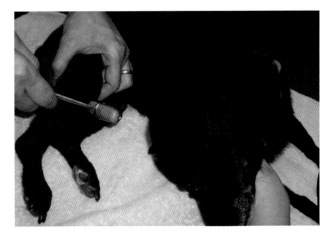

Figure 8.13 Neurological assessment of a patient with vestibular signs.

Table 8.4 Common emergencies

Type of emergency	Details to elicit from the client
Urinary difficulties	Straining noted, color of urine, vocalizing (painful),male or female, history of urinary problems
Toxicity	Product name, type of product, quantity ingested, time frame of ingestion, product package
Vomiting or diarrhea	Productive vomit versus retching, frequency, quantity, consistency, color
Seizure	History, duration, frequency, exposure to toxins, current medications
Trauma	Type of trauma, degree of force, area of trauma, obvious injuries, safe transport instruction

touching the floor. If the communication between the paw and brain are intact, the pet will turn its paw right side up. Reflex assessment will give information regarding the specific neural pathways, and whether or not they are intact (Fig. 8.13, Table 8.4).

Emergency medications

Upon resuscitation efforts, medication can be administered via intravenous (IV), intratracheal (IT), and intracardiac routes. Occasionally, venous access is a challenge and certain medication may be administered via intraperitoneal, intramuscular, and sublingual routes. Classic emergency pharmacology consists of positive inotropes, positive chronotropes, and antiarrhythmics. Oxygen continues to be one of the first-line drugs as the body is hypoxic when in a shock state.

Epinephrine is a positive inotrope that stimulates the myocardium by increasing force and rate: it increases cardiac output, constricts peripheral vessels causing increase in blood pressure, and it also increases blood glucose levels. Dobutamine is similar to epinephrine, yet it causes systemic vasodilation, consequently improving tissue perfusion. Dopamine is also similar to epinephrine, and will dilate the renal arteries when used at low doses, thus improving perfusion to the kidneys. Atropine is an anticholinergic drug used to increase the heart rate (positive chronotropic drug).

Antiarrhythmic agents commonly used include both ventricular and supraventricular antiarrhythmia drugs. Propanolol is a beta blocker that is given to treat ventricular arrhythmias and hypertension. Isoproterenol is a beta-adrenergic positive inotrope and it is used to treat heart blocks, sinus bradycardia, and SSS (sick sinus syndrome). Lidocaine is a local anesthetic that is beneficial in the treatment of ventricular arrhythmias and fibrillation by mode of anesthetizing the heart. Bretylium tosylate and magnesium chloride are older chemical defibrillators used to treat ventricular fibrillation. A newer, more popular replacement is amiodarone, which increases the cardiac action potential duration.

Another key emergency drug used is mannitol. Mannitol is an osmotic diuretic that decreases intracranial pressure (ICP) caused by swelling of the brain. While mannitol is not used in the initial shock resuscitation phase, it should be considered in patients with brain trauma, altered mentation, or postcardiopulmonary arrest (CPA).

In more recent years, vasopressin (antidiuretic hormone, ADH) has gained attention for its use in the treatment of shock. The main effect of vasopressin is peripheral vasoconstriction greater than that of epinephrine during hypoxic and acidotic states. When compared to epinephrine in clinical studies, vasopressin was shown to sustain better vital organ perfusion, thus resulting in a prolonged survival. Patients who received vasopressin were also determined to have better pulmonary gas exchange.

Successful treatment of shock continues to be a major focus, with some studies proving medical advances, if not beneficial medical breakthroughs, in the treatment of shock. Several studies have recently taken place, including the monitoring of global perfusion in efforts to correct occult shock, implementing antioxidant fluids, and developing a new generation of drugs to prevent amplification of the inflammatory process.

In addition to new fluids and medications on the rise, there are new devices to assist with resuscitation. A respiratory impedance threshold device (ITD) is gaining attention in the veterinary community. This device causes a small vacuum to accumulate in the thoracic cavity during inspiration, thus pulling more blood into the heart and increasing cardiac preload (and hopefully cardiac output).

It appears that new shock treatments will be available in the next several years. The main goal in developing these treatments is to prevent a reversible shock state from progressing to an irreversible shock state and improving overall survival. Detection of abnormalities and prevention of deterioration of disease states is the key to success for the patient (Tables 8.5 and 8.6).

Table 8.5 Cardiac compression techniques

Cardiac compression techniques	Benefits/indications
Lateral recumbency	Small, narrow chest
Dorsal recumbency	Large, barrel chest
Cardiac pump	Patients less than 15 lb
Thoracic pump	Patients over 15 lb
Simultaneous ventilation and cardiac compressions (SVCC)	Greater blood flow, pressure, and return
Interposed abdominal compressions (IAC)	Improves venous return and cranial blood flow
Continuous chest compressions	Improves neurological outcome
Open chest compressions	Provides better cerebral and coronary blood flow than external compressions
Active compression and decompression devices	Increased blood flow to the brain, increased survival rates in human studies

Table 8.6 Emergency drug dosing table

Drug	IV dose	Action
Atepamezole (5 mg/mL)	Same dose as Domitor used; can repeat with half dose	Medetomidine reversal
Atropine (0.54 mg/mL)	1 mL/40 lb (up to 0.05 mg/kg)	Parasympatholytic
Bretylol (50 mg/mL)	0.4 mL/10 lb bolus, repeat dose over 10 minute if needed (5–10 mg/kg)	Chemical defibrillator
Dobutamine (12.5 mg/mL)	0.16 mL/lb in 100 mL chamber ran at 1 mL/min (using 10 mcg/kg/min) (2–20 mcg/kg/min)	+Inotrope, systemic vasodilation
Dopamine (40 mg/mL)	0.01 mL/lb in 100 mL chamber ran at 1 mL/min (using 2 mcg/kg/min) (1–10 mcg/kg/min)	+Inotrope, vasoconstriction
Dopram (20 mg/mL)	0.2 mL/lb (2 mg/kg)	Respiratory stimulant
Epinephrine 1:1000 (1 mg/mL)	1 mL/20 lb or 1 mL/10 lb IT (0.1 mg/kg IV; 0.2 mL/kg IT)	+Inotrope, +chronotrope
Hydroxyethyl starch (6% solution)	20 mL/lb rapid IV infusion (20 mL/kg/day;10 mL/kg/day feline dose)	Colloid
Lidocaine 2% (20 mg/mL)	1 mL/20 lb; 1 mL/10 lb fel (2 mg/kg) (0.5 mg/kg feline dose)	Antiarrhythmia (ventricular)
Mannitol 20% (200 mg/mL)	5 mL/lb over 20–30 minutes (0.5 g/kg)	Osmotic diuretic (cerebral edema)
Mg chloride (00 mg/mL)	10 mL over 2 minutes (2 g over 2 minutes)	Chemical defibrillator
Naloxone (0.4 mg/mL)	1 mL/20 lb (0.4 mg/kg)	Opiate antagonist
Sodium bicarbonate 8.4% (1 mEq/mL)	10 mL/20 lb SLOW (1 mEq/kg)	Alkalinizing agent

Chapter references and further reading

J.L. Cornick-Seahorn, S. Marks (1998) Emergency! Treating patients in shock. Veterinary Technician the Complete Journal for the Veterinary Hospital Staff **19**(5): 355-369.

H. Davis (2001) Initial management of the emergent or critically ill patient. Wild West Veterinary Conference.

T. Hackett (2008) Emergency rapid assessment. The National Association of Veterinary Technicians in America Journal **Winter**: 39-43.

J. Keefe (2008) Emergencies: get a grip. International Veterinary Emergency and Critical Care Symposium.

C. Norkus (2008) Management of cardiopulmonary arrest. Veterinary Technician the Complete Journal for the Veterinary Hospital Staff **29**(11): 671-676.

J. Proulx (2003) Cardiopulmonary cerebral resuscitation. American Animal Hospital Association Scientific Program.

R. Scalf (2006) Canine traumatic injury. The National Association of Veterinary Technicians in America Journal **Winter**: 37-42.

M. Schaer (2003) Metabolic and electrolyte emergencies. Western Veterinary Conference.

R. Wells (2008) CPCR: overview and updates. International Veterinary Emergency and Critical Care Symposium.

K. Wuestenberg (2008) Recognition and treatment of shock. International Veterinary Emergency and Critical Care Symposium.

Chapter 9
Harmonizing Hospice Needs

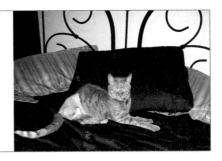

Pet hospice care is an alternative means to managing end stages of life when a natural death is preferred by the owner or until the decision for euthanasia can be made. Hospice care is a palliative therapy, meaning it is not a cure, but an extension of life by treating ailments in the most effective manner while providing comfort and care in terminally ill animals. Veterinary hospice care began in the late 1970s; however, it wasn't until recently that it has become more widely recognized. More and more pet owners consider their pets to be a part of the family. As the movement of human hospice health care has benefited family members of terminally ill individuals, pet hospice care may also provide the same benefits to pet owners. The compassionate and supportive experience of veterinary hospice may help the owner emotionally during the shortened life expectancy.

Home hospice veterinary care is gaining in availability with the help of the human hospice philosophy transferring to pets. The main goal is to comfortably provide supportive care to terminally ill pets while allowing family members to spend quality time caring for them. While the veterinarian and veterinary staff may work with families to provide in-home hospice care, many pets remain in the hospital while decisions are being made by pet owners. The decision of euthanasia is undoubtedly a difficult one. The option of hospice care allows the owner to determine how and when their pet will succumb.

With the human-animal bond continuing to grow stronger, some companion animal hospitals are branching into services for the terminally ill. The pet owner and pet should have a personalized plan developed which consists of the pet's needs, the owner's needs, education, and emotional support. For pet owners who decide against euthanasia or would like to delay euthanasia, hospice care is a means for the pet to live out the rest of their life while under the medical care of veterinarians, technicians, and assistants while also receiving care from their owners and family members (Fig. 9.1).

Family members should be properly trained in husbandry for debilitated animals as well as obtaining basic vital sign parameters such as a heart rate or pulse rate and

Clinical Small Animal Care: Promoting Patient Health through Preventative Nursing, First Edition. Kimm Wuestenberg.
© 2012 John Wiley & Sons, Inc. Published 2012 by John Wiley & Sons, Inc.

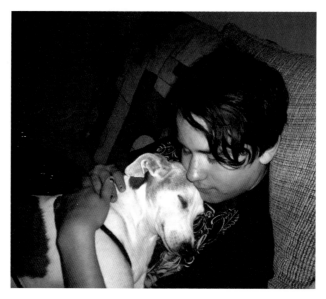

Figure 9.1 The human animal bond.

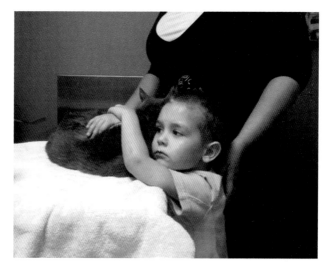

Figure 9.2 Providing veterinary hospice counseling to the family.

assessment, body temperature, and respiratory rate. It is imperative that terminally ill patients are frequently assessed for pain levels and signs of organ failure. Pharmacological intervention plays a major role in hospice care, and although protocol standards have not yet been set, it may be in the near future. Additionally, hygiene and husbandry is an essential aspect of hospice care. Hospice hygienic needs are quite similar to those of the recumbent patient.

The veterinary healthcare team should remain in close contact with the pet owners during hospice. Availability for pain management, nursing care, or euthanasia should be available 24 hours a day. If hospice care is taking place outside of the veterinary practice, home visits by veterinarians, veterinary technicians, or assistants should be arranged on (at least) a daily basis to ensure the pet's medical needs are being met. This visit may also be used as a respite care, where the family members can spend this time tending to their day-to-day responsibilities (Fig. 9.2).

Veterinary hospice care is unique in that it allows pet owners and family members to experience caregiving in the comfort of their home while also experiencing the process of death in an environment other than in-clinic euthanasia. All family members, including children, are encouraged to participate in the care of the terminal patient. Much like the process of performing physical therapy, the loving care involved in hospice care can strengthen or deepen the bond between the pet and family members. Hospice care is a time-consuming service for the veterinary healthcare team and may require additional resources such as psychologists or grief counselors, homeopathic or holistic veterinarians, massage therapists or veterinary chiropractors, pastoral counselors or animal chaplains, and even pet sitters for respite (Fig. 9.3, Table 9.1).

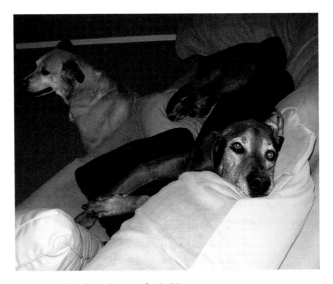

Figure 9.3   Keeping geriatric pets comfortable.

Table 9.1   American Veterinary Medical Association (AVMA) guidelines for hospice care

Family/household dynamics are a consideration when deciding whether veterinary hospice care is appropriate. Veterinarians should counsel clients regarding the severity of their animal's illness or condition and the expected outcome. Clients also should be informed of their responsibilities as well as the services to be provided by the veterinarian.

As with any service, fees should be discussed and agreed upon before hospice service is provided.

(Continued)

Table 9.1 (*Continued*)

Patients should be kept as free from pain as possible and in a sanitary state. Appropriate analgesics may be needed, and, subject to applicable practice acts, the veterinary hospice team should be prepared to train clients in the administration of drugs and other necessary routine care. Clients and caregivers may need to be instructed in the assessment of patients' pain levels and stages of organ system failure. Veterinarians should have contact with clients and patients on a regular and frequent basis. Veterinarians should recognize that this is an emotional and stressful time for clients of terminally ill companion animals and, despite training by the veterinary hospice team, clients may not be able to perform necessary medical treatments in the home setting. Regular visits will allow veterinarians and their staff to assess how clients are coping with treatment protocols.

The veterinary practice must have an appropriate Drug Enforcement Administration and state license, and keep records of all drugs and supplies dispensed.

Veterinary staff should be part of the veterinary hospice team. Insurance coverage for staff must be considered, and should include liability and travel coverage. The latter is important if staff members will be traveling to and from the client's residence.

Clients should be advised, preferably before the animal dies, of their options concerning care of the animal's remains.

In the case of home deaths, clients may need confirmation of death through absence of vital signs or pronouncement of death by the attending veterinarian.

Euthanasia service should be available if the client and veterinarian at any time believe this service is appropriate. If clients are to be present, they should be informed of the events involved in euthanasia prior to their occurrence. Clients may need time alone with the deceased companion animal.

Optimally, veterinary care should be available at all times. This includes after-hours referral for emergency care or advice.

Records must be kept of all interactions with patients and clients, including visits, patient observations, treatments, telephone conversations, and instructions.

A team approach, encompassing professionals in veterinary medicine and psychosocial care is the ideal. The veterinary hospice team should be prepared to recommend that clients contact licensed mental health professionals who are trained and experienced in grief and bereavement.

Approved by the AVMA Executive Board April 2001; reaffirmed April 2007.

Chapter references and further reading

American Veterinary Medical Association. 2007. Guidelines for veterinary hospice care. March 2007. http://www.avma.org/issues/policy/hospice_care.asp

E. Bittel (2008) Quality of life ~ quality of death. First International Symposium on Veterinary Hospice Care, Davis, CA. http://landofpuregold.com/cancer/the-pdfs/quality.pdf

M. Cohan (2005) Euthanasia and pet bereavement. *Veterinary Technician the Complete Journal for the Veterinary Hospital Staff* **26**(10): 706-710.

K. Herzberg (2009) Postoperative nursing care for intervertebral disc disease. *Veterinary Technician the Complete Journal for the Veterinary Hospital Staff* **30**(4): 15-20.

K. Maroccino (2008) Veterinary hospice care: its history and development. *The Latham Letter*. Fall 2008, Volume **XXIX**, No. 4.

R. Sereno (2005) Pain management for cancer patients. *The National Association of Veterinary Technicians in America Journal* **Winter**: 45-50.

R. Timmins (2008) A family veterinarian's perspective on the human-animal bone and hospice care-giving. *The Latham Letter*. Fall 2008, Volume **XXIX**, No. 4.

Section 3

Proper Care of Tubes and Catheters

Chapter 10

Venous and Arterial Catheter Care

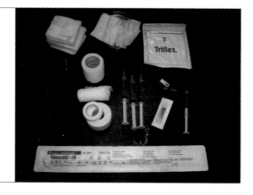

Peripheral intravenous catheters (IVCs) are the most common means of gaining venous access. Peripheral catheters are routinely used in general practice for anesthetic or surgical procedures as well as a means of delivering fluid therapy to ill or injured patients. Although these catheters are routine in practice, it is essential that the practice of caring for these catheters become routine. The typical life span of a peripheral catheter is 3 days, although it is possible to maintain them longer, even up to 5 days. IVCs should be viewed as a direct line to the heart, and thus should be handled as aseptically as possible.

The root of the problem is twofold: first, by securing and bandaging an unclean catheter site, and second, by failing to implement routine care. It is important to recognize that bacteria are attracted to blood. In most cases, blood will contaminate the skin during the initial placement of the catheter, although it is possible (and often a challenge) to place the catheter without a drop of blood spilled. When this blood is not removed from the skin prior to taping and bandaging, a culture medium, in essence, is being created.

The protective catheter bandage should be checked frequently to ensure the bandage is clean and dry. Any time the bandage is wet, it must be changed to prevent infection. It is not uncommon for these bandages to become soiled with vomit, urine, blood, or fluid solutions. The catheter should be flushed with a heparinized saline every 8 hours. When attachments such as connectors or extension sets become engulfed with blood or blood clots, the sets should be changed and replaced with new connection sets. The decision to cover an IVC or to leave it visible is up to the practices of the facility and the nursing personnel. Bandages can range from a simple porous tape wrap to a modified Robert Jones covering using cast padding, roll gauze, and flexible bandage (Figs. 10.1 and 10.2).

At least once every 24 hours, the catheter bandage should be removed and the insertion site observed for erythema, phlebitis, discharge, or other signs of infection. If the

Clinical Small Animal Care: Promoting Patient Health through Preventative Nursing, First Edition. Kimm Wuestenberg.
© 2012 John Wiley & Sons, Inc. Published 2012 by John Wiley & Sons, Inc.

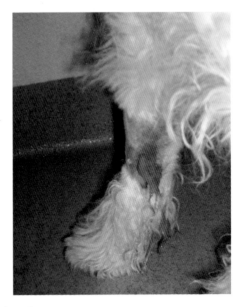

Figure 10.1 IV catheter abscess.

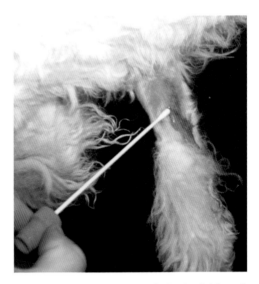

Figure 10.2 Obtaining sample for culture. Result: *Escherichia coli.*

catheter site displays signs of infection, it should be removed and replaced in a separate site if the catheter is still required. The site should be disinfected and retaped if soiled with blood, urine, or other material. The toes should be examined for swelling, coolness, pallor, or other signs of poor circulation. The area proximal to the catheter should be observed, noting any swelling or pain to the touch, indicating lack of patency or possible phlebitis or infection (Fig. 10.3). Once the catheter site has been disinfected and thoroughly evaluated, it may be rebandaged. If the entire paw is to be bandaged, bandaging

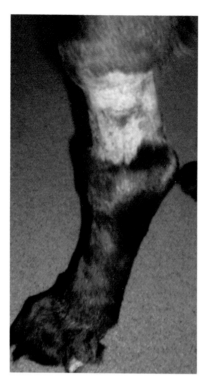

Figure 10.3 Phlebitis and edema at an IV catheter site.

should begin at the toes, moving proximally. It is recommended to use a light gauze wrap and then secure with a tertiary layer such as a flexible bandage material. The extension ports and sets should be anchored to prevent dislodgement, either from the catheter or of the catheter itself (Fig. 10.4).

Maintaining the central venous catheter

Central venous catheters have a wide variety of use in veterinary medicine, from administering parenteral nutrition, to measuring central venous pressure (CVP), or are simply used as a blood collection port in patients requiring serial blood tests with atraumatic collection. Central venous catheters can remain in place longer than peripheral IVCs provided that proper care of the catheter has been practiced. These catheters come in single, double, and multiple lumens, which allows for multipurpose use from one centrally placed catheter.

While central venous catheter use is particularly beneficial for many critically ill or injured patients and those requiring long-term hospitalization, there are instances where they are contraindicated. For instance, a patient with head trauma suffering from poor blood drainage from the cerebral venous system may acquire cerebral edema if a central venous catheter is placed in the jugular vein. Additionally, it may be safer for a patient with a severe coagulopathy to receive serial peripheral venipuncture for

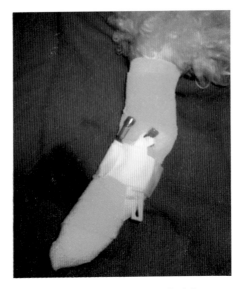

Figure 10.4 Securing the catheter with bandage material.

Table 10.1 Blood sampling steps using a central venous catheter

1. Flush catheter with 1-2 mL of heparinized saline
2. Remove 3 mL blood, save syringe
3. Remove desired blood sample
4. Inject heparin/blood solution in small or anemic patients
5. Flush catheter with 2-3 mL of heparinized saline

Table 10.2 CVP procedure

Normal range 0-5 mmH$_2$O

Jugular central venous catheter is required

Manometer is held at level of heart

Steps:

1. Turn off to manometer (catheter patency)
2. Turn off to patient (filling the manometer)
3. Ensure no air or bubbles are in manometer
4. Turn off to fluid bag
5. Manometer fluid will drop to CVP reading
6. Fluid will slightly fluctuate as the heart beats

testing rather than risk severe hemorrhage from central venous catheter placement. In the same respect, patients in a hypercoagulable state, such as immune-mediated hemolytic anemia or a protein-losing nephropathy, are at greater risk for developing a pulmonary thromboembolism or suffering from thrombosis of the vena cava (Tables 10.1 and 10.2).

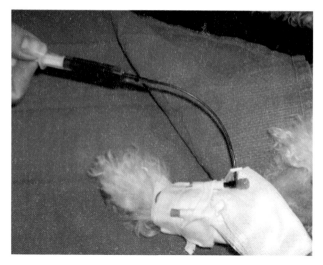

Figure 10.5 Blood collection using a central venous catheter.

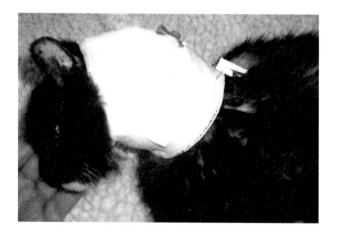

Figure 10.6 Central venous catheter placed using the jugular vein.

   Maintaining the central venous catheter consists of typical venous access site inspection for erythema, phlebitis, or signs of thrombosis or other signs of infection. In addition, due to the large diameter of the catheter, there is often more bleeding and bruising at these catheter sites. It is recommended to unwrap the catheter bandage material instead of cutting the bandage material because it is possible to cut the catheter, sending it into systemic circulation. There is usually a portion of the catheter hidden beneath the bandage material, so proper labeling of the catheter is recommended (Figs. 10.5-10.7).

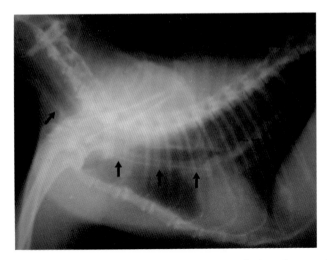

Figure 10.7 Radiograph confirmation of central venous catheter placement.

Intraosseous catheter care and maintenance

Intraosseous (IO) catheters have been used in human medicine since 1922, yet they are often underutilized in veterinary medicine. An IO catheter can be lifesaving during an emergency where venous access is difficult to establish or maintain due to collapse. Commercially available IO catheters may be used for placement; however, spinal needles and hypodermic needles are also acceptable for use as IO catheters. Fluid therapy, medications, and even blood products can be delivered via the IO route, in most cases at the same rate as intravenous (IV) administration. In fact, IO access provides a faster delivery than peripheral venous access and the same rate of delivery as central venous access. This efficiency, combined with ease of placement and noncollapsible qualities, makes these catheters invaluable in an emergency.

Additionally, IO catheters provide quick, easy venous access for neonates, small animals, and many exotic species. These particular catheters are not recommended in adults or large breeds because adult bones contain more yellow marrow than red marrow. There is also a higher level of difficulty in penetrating through bone in these cases. IO catheters should be avoided in bones which have sustained a fracture or previous IO catheter; if there is an infection or wound at the proposed insertion site; or in situations where placement landmarks are not detectable, such as edema.

IO catheters are typically placed in the greater trochanter (intertrochanteric fossa) of the femur. Other sites include the large trochanter of the humerus, the diaphysis of the ulna, the tuberosity of the tibia, and the iliac portion of the pelvis. These catheters, which have virtually been placed in a bone, will be able to deliver into circulation due to a network of venous sinusoids in the medullary canal that lead to the nutrient vessels that flow directly into systemic venous circulation.

When placed and maintained properly, the risks of complications are minimal. Risk data for human IO catheter complications are at a rate of less than 1%. Nonetheless, there are complications that should be understood in order to appropriately monitor the patient with IO access. Placement risks include fracture of the bone, epiphyseal damage, which may lead to a bone growth disturbance, damage to the sciatic nerve, and extravasation.

With regard to clinically monitoring the patient with an established IO catheter, complications such as pain, osteomyelitis, infection, and dislodgement of the catheter may occur. A more serious complication well documented in human medicine but rarely noted in veterinary medicine is acute compartment syndrome (ACS). ACS typically occurs when extravasation (either through bone penetration, fracture, or through the foramen of a nutrient vessel, etc.) has caused an increased pressure in osseofascial (bone and muscle) compartments and decreases capillary perfusion. The end result is cellular hypoxia, muscle ischemia, and tissue death. Clinical signs of ACS include edema, pain, paralysis, paresis, cold limb, or an absent pulse. Current therapeutics for ACS is limited to emergency surgical fasciotomy or amputation. The use of osmotic diuretics is a therapeutic possibility that has undergone recent investigation in human medicine.

Maintenance of the IO catheter will be a short-lived experience as these catheters are typically recommended for only 24- to 48-hour use; however, a 96-hour life span is possible with proper care and patient consideration. IO catheters can be painful for the patient and replacing it with another means of venous access is recommended as soon as possible. However, while the catheter is in place, maintenance is very similar to peripheral catheter care. The insertion site should be kept clean and covered if possible, although these areas are often difficult to bandage. The catheter may be sutured to the patient directly, or with "butterfly" tape tabs. As with all catheters, keeping the region free of blood and other secretions is essential in preventing an infection. The catheter site should be flushed with heparinized saline and disinfected at least every 24 hours. Tubing (T-ports, extension sets, etc.) should be replaced as needed. The patient should be monitored for pain, swelling, or signs of infection (Fig. 10.8).

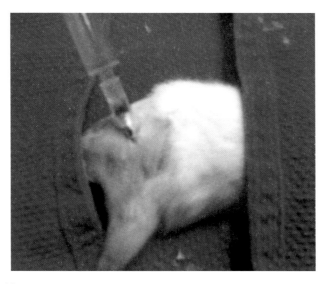

Figure 10.8 IO access.

Venous access ports

Venous access ports or devices are used for patients receiving long-term fluid or drug administration, such as oncology patients receiving chemotherapy or chronic renal patients in need of fluid therapy on a routine basis. These devices are generally reserved for long-term conditions or for those patients with difficult-to-access veins. Venous access ports are beneficial in that they reduce stress and anxiety associated with repetitive catheter placement, they are painless once in place, and they provide a means of quick venous access (either for blood collection or medication and fluid delivery). Another benefit of venous access ports is that nutritional therapy can be delivered as they reside in a large vessel, most commonly the jugular vein. Venous access ports are surgically placed while the patient is under anesthesia. Care of the venous access port involves cleaning and aseptically preparing the injection site prior to use and completely flushing the device with heparinized saline after use to ensure patency. Occasionally a local anesthetic may be needed while using the port if the needle insertion will be over a considerable amount of time and the patient is in discomfort.

Maintaining the arterial catheter

Arterial access is often reserved for direct blood pressure monitoring and serial blood gas analysis and is not used as a route of fluid therapy. It is an invasive procedure, with the dorsal metatarsal artery being the most common site of catheter placement. Arterial blood gases are an essential part of diagnosing and managing oxygen and acid–base status disorders. Arterial catheters are generally reserved for critically ill respiratory or metabolic patients.

Arterial catheters should be flushed with at least 3 mL of heparinized saline every 2 hours. The catheter and attachments should be kept clean, free of blood and other debris. The catheter site should be monitored for signs of infection such as phlebitis, erythema, or edema. The catheter should be removed if signs of infection occur (Table 10.3).

Table 10.3 Quick reference of venous access catheter maintenance

Catheter type	General maintenance
Peripheral	• Keep bandage clean and dry • Strip down, rewrap, flush with heplock and disinfect every 24 hours • Replace T-port as needed • Remove catheter if signs of infection
Central venous	• Keep bandage clean and dry • Strip down, re-wrap, flush with heplock and disinfect every 24 hours • Flush with a heplock every 6 hours if not used for fluid therapy • Replace T-port as needed • Remove catheter if there are signs of infection • Watch for swelling (facial or distal extremities if saphenous/femoral)

Table 10.3 *(Continued)*

Catheter type	General maintenance
Arterial	• Flush with at least 3 mL of heplock every 2 hours • Keep art line clean, free of blood • Monitor for signs of infection
IO	• IO catheter care is same as IVC care • Keep site clean and dry • Flush with heplock and disinfect every 24 hours • Replace T-port as needed • Remove catheter if signs of infection • Watch for swelling • Recommended to replace with IV access as soon as possible

Chapter references and further reading

S. Bateman (2003a) Placing central venous catheters. Western Veterinary Conference.

S. Bateman (2003b) Tips for IV care. Western Veterinary Conference.

T. Crowe (2003) Vascular access techniques. *The National Association of Veterinary Technicians in America Journal* **Spring**: 45-48.

S. Erickson (2008) Thoracocentesis, chest tube management and arterial sampling. International Veterinary Emergency and Critical Care Symposium.

T. Hacket (2003) Vascular access tips in cats. Western Veterinary Conference.

D. Heath (1998) Lifeline to recovery: intravenous catheterization techniques. *Veterinary Technician the Complete Journal for the Veterinary Hospital Staff* **19**(10): 614-621.

J. Keefe (2008) Central lines, female urinary catheterization, N/G tube placement. International Veterinary Emergency and Critical Care Symposium.

O. Lanz (2003) Long term vascular access. Western Veterinary Conference.

D. Reeder (2008) Arterial blood pressure monitoring. *Veterinary Technician the Complete Journal for the Veterinary Hospital Staff* **29**(8): 478-483.

N. Royer (1998) Placing a catheter in a dorsal pedal vein. *Veterinary Technician the Complete Journal for the Veterinary Hospital Staff* **19**(1): 58-59.

H. Ruess-Lamki (2008) The fine art of art(erial) lines. International Veterinary Emergency and Critical Care Symposium.

K. Wuestenberg (2008) Intraosseous catheters, abdominocentesis, gastric lavage and neonatal resuscitation. International Veterinary Emergency and Critical Care Symposium.

Chapter 11
Indwelling Urinary Catheter Care and Maintenance

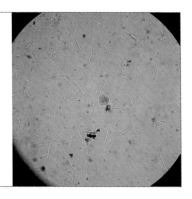

Urinary catheters which are placed for long-term use require special attention by the nursing staff to ensure that patient health is not compromised. In addition, monitoring the urine output will give valuable information about the patient such as indications of urinary tract infection, fluid overload, and kidney function. Proper urinary catheter maintenance and patient nursing care will help reduce the risk of nosocomial infections and complications associated with indwelling urinary catheters. Clinical scenarios where indwelling urinary catheter placement is indicated include (but are not limited to) conditions such as urinary tract obstruction, the critical care patient (monitoring perfusion and renal function), recumbent or paralyzed patients, and patients with neurogenic bladder dysfunction.

Daily catheter care

The urinary catheter should be thoroughly examined at least every 2 hours to ensure that the catheter and collection set is patent, the patient is producing urine, and the urinary catheter is clean and free of fecal material, vomitus, or any other debris. Females are at higher risk for fecal contamination of the urinary catheter due to the external genitalia being in close proximity to the rectum. The patient's skin surrounding the urinary catheter should also be examined for signs of infection. Urine can leak around the catheter and soil the skin, leading to scald and infection.

Every 8 hours the catheter should be flushed with 5–10 mL of sterile saline to ensure it is patent. Blood clots and other flocculent material may obstruct the catheter, indicating the catheter should be replaced. The catheter and external genitalia should also be disinfected with a light povidone-iodine solution or 0.05% chlorhexidine solution every 8 hours. Placing an antimicrobial ointment at the catheter site is strongly recommended as cleaning alone may lead to bacteriuria.

Clinical Small Animal Care: Promoting Patient Health through Preventative Nursing, First Edition.
Kimm Wuestenberg.
© 2012 John Wiley & Sons, Inc. Published 2012 by John Wiley & Sons, Inc.

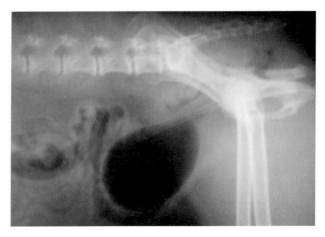

Figure 11.1 Proper urinary catheter positioning.

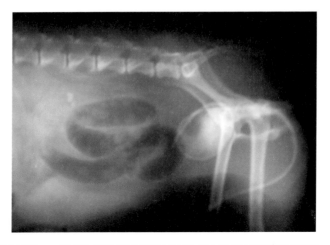

Figure 11.2 Improper urinary catheter placement due to measuring error.

Urinary catheters may remain in place for 3-4 days. If infection is suspected (fever, purulent discharge, sediment exhibiting white blood cells [WBCs] and bacteria, strong urine odor, etc.), the urinary catheter should be removed. If warranted, the patient may have a new urinary catheter placed (Figs. 11.1 and 11.2).

Daily collection set care

The recommended standard of care for patients with an indwelling urinary catheter is the use of a closed urinary collection system. Collection sets will help reduce the risk of urinary tract infections as well as help maintain patient hygiene and more specifically, decrease the likelihood of urine scalding of the patients' skin.

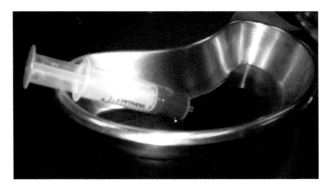

Figure 11.3   Gross exam of methemoglobinuria.

The collection set should always be kept below the level of the patient. This will prevent the urine from traveling from the collection set back into the bladder (retrograde urine flow). The collection set and lines should be changed every 24 hours and replaced with a new collection system.

Urine collecting in the set should be evaluated and removed from the bag every 2 hours. Ports already existing in the collection set may be used to remove the urine. Alternately, a three-way stopcock may be placed on the line and used as a means of urine removal. A gross examination of the urine should be performed and documented in the medical record. Key points in the gross examination include the description of color, turbidity, odor or volume—including the detection of any changes in these areas. It is also recommended to perform a urinalysis every 24–48 hours to monitor for signs of urinary infection. If an infection is suspected, a urine sample may be taken from the collection bag, line, or the catheter itself and submitted for culture and sensitivity testing (Figs. 11.3–11.6).

Commercial urinary collection systems are available; however, urinary collection systems may be made in the clinic using fluid bags, administration sets, and extension sets. The administration flow dial and any closure apparatus are to be removed or altered in a manner that keeps the line open and free from occlusion at all times. These items may be removed from the line or secured open with porous tape. If new fluid bags (emptied) and lines are not being used for the set, then it is recommended to sterilize the collections systems prior to use (gas sterilization). The addition of 3% hydrogen peroxide (5–10 mL) to the collection bag can help reduce the risk of urinary infections; however this should not be used in cases exhibiting hematuria, as the gas created when hydrogen peroxide encounters blood can obstruct the urine flow. It should be noted that hydrogen peroxide addition to collection sets may also alter urinalysis results (Figs. 11.7–11.9).

Patient nursing

Patients with an indwelling urinary catheter should always have an Elizabethan collar (E-collar) in place to prevent the patient from chewing, grooming, or disconnecting the

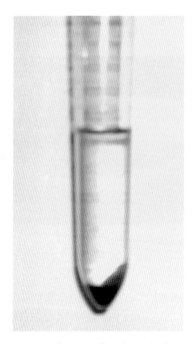

Figure 11.4 Centrifuged urine sample revealing hematuria.

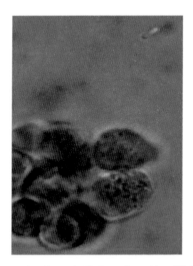

Figure 11.5 Microscopic examination of WBC cast and bacilli found in urine sediment.

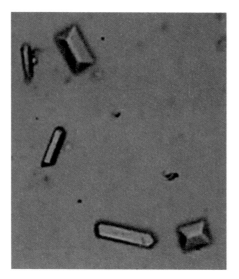

Figure 11.6 Struvite crystals.

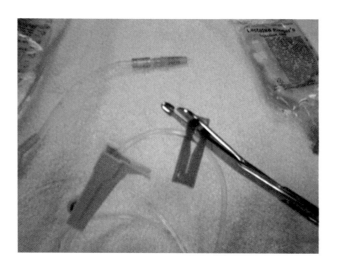

Figure 11.7 Removing administration clamp.

catheter or collection system. The lines should be checked frequently to ensure urine flow. It is not uncommon for the patient to circle, pace, or ambulate in a manner that obstructs the flow. If the patient has other tubing in place (feeding tube, intravenous catheter, nasal oxygen, etc.) the lines may become entangled, causing obstruction of flow. The remaining external urinary catheter and proximal collection set line should be taped to the tail (parallel) to help prevent inadvertent removal of the urinary catheter through patient movement. In patients lacking a tail, the urinary catheter and collection tubing may be taped to one of the rear extremities.

Quantifying fluid input and fluid output is one of the most important aspects of patient monitoring. The use of a urinary catheter is a key tool in monitoring urine output.

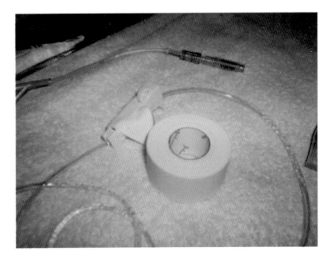

Figure 11.8 Securing the flow dial in "open" position.

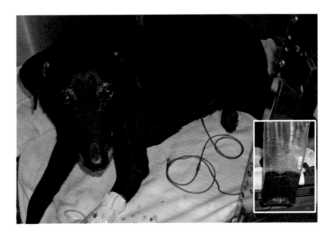

Figure 11.9 Complete urinary collection set using intravenous administration set and fluid bag.

Normal urine output is 1–2 mL/kg/h. Volumes less than this rate are considered oliguric and can indicate poor perfusion and/or impaired renal function. Volumes which are greater than 1–2 mL/kg/h can indicate diuresis or patient volume overload. It is not uncommon for posturinary tract obstruction patients to exhibit diuresis, and special attention to fluid balances should be taken to ensure the patient is not overhydrated. In addition, patients with low blood pressure may progress into acute renal failure, exhibited by oliguria (0.25–0.5 mL/kg/h) or anuria (no urine production). Monitoring the urine production is essential in preventing patient deterioration in these cases.

Miscellaneous urinary tubes

Occasionally the need arises for a patient to require a nontraditional means of eliminating urine. Patients with cancers of the bladder, urethra, or genitourinary region may benefit from a cystotomy tube. A cystotomy tube is surgically placed and, much like the gastrotomy tube, provides a patent pathway to the exterior of the patient where the tube can be handled by caregivers. The cystotomy tube requires that a caregiver uncap the tube and allow the patient's bladder to be voided of urine every 4–8 hours. This tube should also be inspected and disinfected at least once a day.

Another alternative urinary catheter is one which resides in the ureter. Ureteral catheters can be utilized for disease states involving the bladder, urethra, or genitourinary regions such as in prostatic cancers. Additionally, when obstruction of the distal ureter is present, a ureteral catheter can help prevent hydronephrosis and provide a means of eliminating urine. Ureteral catheters require absolute securing and careful handling of the external portion of the catheter. The catheter should be covered or bandaged and secured in a manner that the patient will not dislodge the catheter. The insertion site should be examined and disinfected at least once a day (Tables 11.1 and 11.2).

Table 11.1 Urinary catheter care maintenance

Quick reference			
Task	**Includes**	**Frequency**	**Rationale**
Patient hygiene and catheter patency	Keeping skin clean, observing collection set for urine production and flow; catheter replacement if necessary	As often as possible; every 2 hours at minimum	Prevent infection, skin scalding, obstruction of urine flow
Flush and disinfect catheter site	Flush with 5–10 mL of sterile saline; disinfect with povidone-iodine or chlorhexidine, place antimicrobial ointment	Every 8 hours; more frequent if indicated	Prevent nosocomial infection and ensure catheter patency
Urine gross exam and documentation	Color, odor, turbidity, and volume; balancing fluid ins/outs	Every 2 hours: more frequent if indicated	Detect urinary infection, overhydration, or poor perfusion/kidney dysfunction
Change collection system	Removal of collection bag, line, and extension sets and placement of new system	Every 24 hours; more frequent if indicated	Prevent nosocomial infection; maintain accurate current gross exam
Perform urinalysis	Gross exam, chemistry, urine specific gravity (USG), and sediment examination; remove or replace catheter as indicated	Every 24–48 hours: more frequent if indicated	Identify signs of infections or changes in patient status (glycosuria, USG, cylindruria, etc.)

Table 11.2 Urinary catheter troubleshooting guide

Problem	Considerations
Urine not flowing into collection set	• Make sure collection lines are not kinked or twisted, flush to ensure patency • Disconnect collection set and flush catheter (checking patency) • Confirm catheter placement (radiograph) • Measure the patients' blood pressure (ensuring adequate perfusion, detecting oliguric or anuric renal failure) • Evaluate patient status (i.e., multiple organ dysfunction syndrome [MODS])
Significant amount of urine leakage around catheter	• Consider size of catheter; replacement may be indicated • Follow insufflation guidelines (Foley catheters) • Flush catheter (ensure patency) • Perform cytology of fluid to rule out purulent discharge • Arrange a disposable bed pad or towel to protect the patient from soiling skin
Patient chewing on/ licking catheter or collection line	• Place larger E-collar • Consider chew deterrent spray • Place towel over collection line
Catheter slipping out of place (moving distally from original position)	• Resuture • Anchor to tail with tape • Confirm catheter placement (radiograph)
Patient discomfort	• Consider analgesics • Resuture or retape catheter if too much tension being placed • Observe for signs of infection

Chapter references and further reading

A. Battaglia-Lawrence (1998) Urinary catheter placement in male dogs. *Veterinary Technician the Complete Journal for the Veterinary Hospital Staff* **19**(9): 570-573.

J. Keefe (2008) Central lines, female urinary catheterization, N/G tube placement. International Veterinary Emergency and Critical Care Symposium.

S. Okumura (2005) Urine collection techniques. *Veterinary Technician the Complete Journal for the Veterinary Hospital Staff* **26**(10): 720-725.

K. Stafford (2004) Enhanced radiographic studies. *Veterinary Technician the Complete Journal for the Veterinary Hospital Staff* **25**(6): 384-393.

Chapter 12
Feeding Tube Care

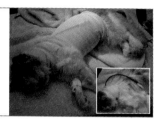

For the seriously ill or injured patient, nutrition is essential to provide basic nutrients and energy. Good nutrition improves the likelihood of recovery as illness creates a state of hypermetabolism and subsequent catabolism. Negative energy balances can result in skeletal and smooth muscle weakness, a disruption of the gastrointestinal mucosal barrier, gastrointestinal ileus, and weakening of the immune system. The overall consensus in meeting the nutritional requirements of ill or injured patients is to utilize the gut if it works.

There are several means of delivering nutrition in an anorectic patient. Orogastric tube feeding is typically reserved for neonates and is an intermittent procedure without the requirement of indwelling tube care (Figs. 12.1 and 12.2). Nasogastric (NG) and naso-esophageal (NE) tubes are utilized for short-term feedings while esophagostomy (EG) and gastrostomy tubes can be used for longer periods of time, allowing the patient to return home with the owner administering the feedings. Other feeding tubes used are jejunostomy and duodenostomy tubes. These tubes, however, are primarily reserved for use in the critically ill hospitalized patient.

NG and NE tubes

NG and NE feeding tubes are utilized for short-term nutritional delivery (typically less than 7 days). The tube is placed in the nostril and advanced into the esophagus or stomach after premeasuring the appropriate distance. These feeding tubes have a smaller diameter than other conventional feeding tubes, thus requiring liquid diets.

NG and NE tubes are often used in patients with increased nutritional requirements, recent anorexia (less than 5 days), or in the event of anticipated anorexia (full mouth extraction). They are easily placed and maintained for patients who do not tolerate oral feedings. Additionally, medication can be administered via NG and NE tubes.

Clinical Small Animal Care: Promoting Patient Health through Preventative Nursing, First Edition.
Kimm Wuestenberg.
© 2012 John Wiley & Sons, Inc. Published 2012 by John Wiley & Sons, Inc.

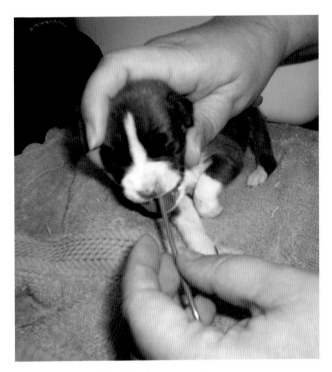

Figure 12.1 Passing an orogastric tube in a neonate.

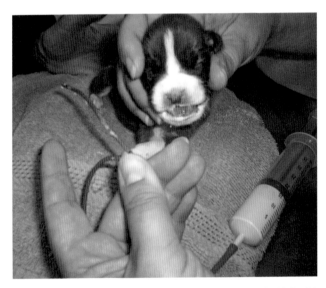

Figure 12.2 Removal of the tube after feeding. Note the tube is kinked to prevent aspiration of contents into the lungs.

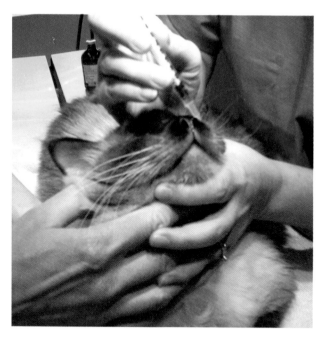

Figure 12.3 Local anesthetic placed into the nasal passages to ease the passing of the tube.

There are instances where it is not recommended to use NG or NE tubes. Some conditions include, but are not limited to, uncontrollable vomiting, nasal cavity fracture, rhinitis, loss of the gag reflex, and altered mentation. Patients with brain, esophageal, pharyngeal, or biliary tract surgery or trauma are not suitable for NG/NE tube placement.

Complications which may arise often result from overfeeding. Overfeeding may result in reflux or vomiting, which may result in an array of events from vomiting and chewing the tube itself to aspiration pneumonia. Epistaxis or sinusitis can also occur, as well as skin infections at the site where the tubes are secured.

These tubes typically are low maintenance. The tube entry site should be kept clean and free of secretions or food. Dermal infections can occur when contact points are left unclean. Some patients may attempt to dislodge the tubes, therefore placement of an Elizabethan collar may be necessary.

Prior to each feeding, the tube should be aspirated to remove any residual stomach juices. After each feeding, the tube should be flushed with water to prevent food from creating a blockage within the tube. If an occlusion does occur, attempts to clear the tube may be made by flushing with warm water (Figs. 12.3-12.5).

EG tube care

EG tubes are often utilized when longer periods of assisted nutrition are needed. These tubes are generally well tolerated and can remain in place anywhere from 1 week to 3

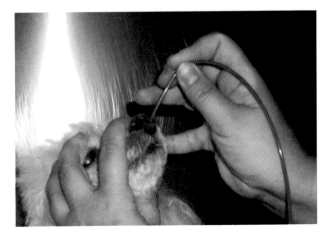

Figure 12.4 Pressing the nose dorsally will open the passageway, easing placement.

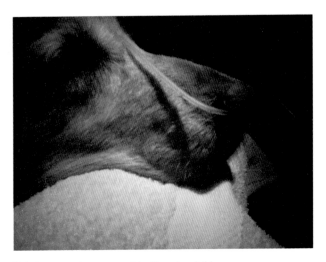

Figure 12.5 NG tubes can be secured in the alar fold.

months at the very most. Esophageal feeding tubes are indicated when nutritional delivery is suspected to last longer than 1 week. These tubes are appropriate for patients suffering from oral cavity or pharyngeal disorders so long as gastrointestinal function is adequate. Like the NE tubes, they should not be used in patients with delayed gastric emptying or uncontrollable vomiting. In addition, they should not be used in patients with esophageal disorders or with recent biliary surgery.

Maintenance of the EG tube involves daily evaluation of the insertion site for signs of infection. The protective covering (usually stockinet) should be changed every 3–5 days or sooner if soiled. Like the NE tube, the tube must be aspirated prior to use and flushed with water after use. It is recommended to wait 24 hours after placement before feedings are implemented (Figs. 12.6 and 12.7).

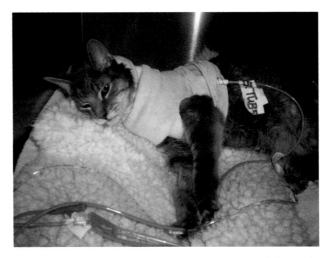

Figure 12.6 EG tube in a geriatric patient, Maddie, who is receiving a slow continuous rate infusion (CRI) of a nutritional supplement diet.

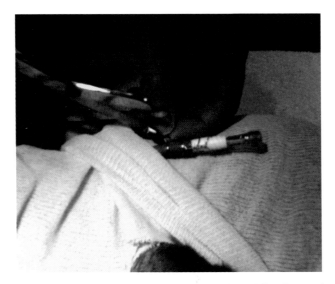

Figure 12.7 Securing an EG tube to be used for intermittent feedings using surgical steel.

Gastrostomy tubes

Gastrostomy tubes are indicated when assisted feeding is expected to last at least 2 weeks, but can be used for several months. Like the EG tube, they can allow for home feedings but feedings should be sustained for the first 12–24 hours after initial placement. These tubes are placed either via endoscope, laparotomy, or percutaneously. Some patients with gastrotomy tubes may require an Elizabethan collar to prevent licking of the site or chewing of the tube. The tube insertion site should be examined on a daily basis, aseptically handled, and disinfected. The dressing–again the stockinet is typically used–should be changed every 3-5 days or sooner if soiling occurs. Like the other indwelling feeding tubes, the stomach contents should be aspirated prior to feeding and the tube flushed with water after the feeding.

Miscellaneous tubes

Jejunostomy and duodenostomy tube insertion sites should be routinely evaluated for position as well as for signs of infection. Nutritional delivery through these tubes is usually through a constant rate infusion of a liquid diet. It is of utmost importance that the intravenous fluid delivery set and nutritional feeding delivery sets are properly and accurately attached to the correct port. Allowing the enteral nutrition to be delivered intravenously can prove to be a fatal error. It is recommended to clearly label all lines leading to the patient to prevent errors such as this from happening (Fig. 12.8).

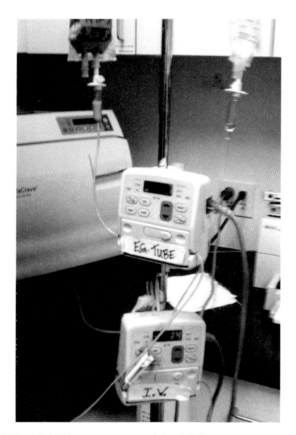

Figure 12.8 Labeling fluid therapy pump and food delivery pump.

Chapter references and further reading

J. Keefe (2008) Central lines, female urinary catheterization, N/G tube placement. International Veterinary Emergency and Critical Care Symposium.

P. Mullane (1998) Practical neonatal care: tube feeding. *Veterinary Technician the Complete Journal for the Veterinary Hospital Staff* **19**(8): 532–535.

J. Proulx (2003) Critical care nutrition II. Western Veterinary Conference.

D. Twedt (2003) Enteral tube feeding. American Animal Hospital Association Scientific Program.

B. Womack (2003) Providing nutritional support to critical care patients. *Veterinary Technician the Complete Journal for the Veterinary Hospital Staff* **24**(6): 376–386.

A. Wortinger (2005) The ins and outs of feeding tubes. *Veterinary Technician the Complete Journal for the Veterinary Hospital Staff* **26**(1): 11–22.

D. Zoran (2003) Enteral nutrition for anorectic cats. Western Veterinary Conference.

Chapter 13
Nasal Oxygen Catheter Care

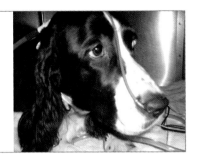

There are several effective ways of administering oxygen to the veterinary patient. Each delivery method comes with advantages and disadvantages which are taken into consideration when determining each individual patient's oxygen therapy needs. Clinical methods of oxygen delivery are discussed further in both the cardiac and respiratory sections as well as in the emergency response section.

Nasal oxygen insufflation is a beneficial therapeutic for many conditions, particularly anemia, cardiogenic disease, lung parenchymal disease, and pleural space disease. Uses also include (but are not limited to) toxicities, central nervous system trauma, and ventilation-perfusion mismatching. These catheters, or cannulas, can be used long term with usually minimal patient discomfort. Nasal oxygen tubes are easily placed and allow for hands-on patient nursing while oxygen is continuously delivered.

Although red rubber catheters are most often used for oxygen insufflation, twin-bore oxygen sets made for human use may be utilized. Due to the potential for dislodgement, patients using a human oxygen set should be restricted to those with minimal activity. Red rubber catheters are most commonly stapled or sutured into place. It is important to ensure the patients' comfort with appropriate placement and minimal tension at the site of attachment. If the patient is uncomfortable, they are more likely to attempt to dislodge the cannula. An Elizabethan collar will help reduce the risk of dislodgement as long as the patient allows for it. In addition, the oxygen system tubing may be secured to the patient with bandage material. This will help prevent the weight or pull of the tubing from dislodging the catheter.

Humidifiers are recommended if nasal insufflation is to last longer than 2 hours. Dry oxygen can cause an increase in secretion viscosity, cause mucociliary dysfunction, and degenerate respiratory epithelium, all of which may increase the risk of a respiratory infection in the patient. In addition, dry oxygen can dehydrate the nasal mucosa and cause discomfort to the patient and, in some instances, cause epistaxis. Oxygen humidification systems create an ideal humidity of 30%–40%. The humidification systems contain a capillary tube that reaches to the bottom of the system container. Bubbles are then formed, and as they rise to the surface, pick up water vapor, which can be delivered to the patient. Humidifiers should always be kept in an upright position to ensure that water does not enter the oxygen pathway to the patient. General

Clinical Small Animal Care: Promoting Patient Health through Preventative Nursing, First Edition. Kimm Wuestenberg.
© 2012 by John Wiley & Sons, Inc. Published 2012 by John Wiley & Sons, Inc.

Table 13.1 Nasal oxygen delivery rates

Weight (in kg)	FiO$_2$ of 30%-50% (L/min)	FiO$_2$ of 50%-75% (L/min)	FiO$_2$ of 75%-100% (L/min)
0-10	0.5-1	1-2	3-5
10-20	1-2	3-5	>5
20-40	3-5	>5	>5

Oxygen flow rate depends on desired O$_2$ percentage and patient body weight. Higher flow rates mean greater risk of complications.

Table 13.2 Troubleshooting guide

Problem	Potential solutions
Dry nasal mucosa or epistaxis	Decrease oxygen flow rate; alternate tube placement to opposite nasal passage; consider the use of bilateral insufflation
Decreased oxygen delivery to the patient	Check all tubes (catheter, oxygen tubing to humidifier, oxygen line to oxygen source) for occlusions; check oxygen supply
Water in the oxygen tube	Check humidifier, ensure it is in upright position
Patient displays signs of dyspnea or poor oxygenation	Evaluate the oxygen delivery system; evaluate the patient based on clinical condition

maintenance of the humidifier requires replacing the water on a daily basis. It is recommended to use distilled water.

Although nasal oxygen catheters can be used long term (up to 1-2 weeks), the catheter itself should be replaced every 48-72 hours, alternating with the opposite nostril to help prevent patient discomfort due to nasal mucosa irritation. It's also important to routinely check the catheter attachment sites and clean any debris, particularly near the alar folds, which may contribute to dermal irritation or infection.

At times, bilateral nasal oxygen tubes are placed. Insufflation of both nasal passages allows for higher flow rates to be obtained while reducing patient discomfort. A study published in 2002 showed that FiO$_2$ and PaO$_2$ rates were the same whether the oxygen was delivered via one tube or two tubes. The study showed that the benefit of utilizing bilateral nasal cannulas was the patient comfort level that was achieved. Although the use of bilateral catheters may not change delivery values, it may help the patient be more tolerable when high flow rates are required. Special care should be taken when using bilateral oxygen catheters, as prolonged administration of oxygen at high flow rates can cause oxygen toxicity in the patient (Tables 13.1 and 13.2).

Chapter references and further reading

E. Mazzaferro (2003) Oxygen therapy. American Animal Hospital Association Scientific Program.

Chapter 14
Tracheostomy Tube Care

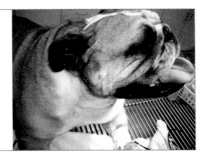

Tracheotomies are typically performed in emergency situations; however, they are also placed as a palliative tool to improve quality of life in some cases where the upper airways are obstructed (tumors, for instance). In the emergent patient, a large-bore peripheral intravenous catheter can be inserted into the trachea and oxygen attached to the catheter (transtracheal catheter). This is a temporary procedure, used while awaiting a tracheotomy.

Once the tracheotomy has been performed, a tracheostomy tube will be placed, creating a temporary or permanent opening depending on the nature of disease. Commercially available tracheostomy tubes are available with introducers, inflatable cuffs, or without a cuff and with interchangeable filter inserts or cannulas. Alternatively, a clear endotracheal tube can be revised to act as a tracheostomy tube, although soft, pliable material is preferred.

The tracheostomy tube is sutured in place and should be secondarily anchored around the neck by umbilical tape and then bandaged with a sterile wound dressing and light wrap. The bandage should be changed on a daily basis or sooner if soiling occurs. The surgical site should be disinfected and observed for signs of infection during this time. The recommended disinfectant solution is a 50:50 mixture of hydrogen peroxide and either sterile water or sterile saline. The tracheotomy site and tracheostomy tube and components should be handled aseptically and sterile gauze placed in between the tube collar and skin to prevent pressure. Additionally, immediate observations should be made for any signs of hemorrhage or emphysema, either subcutaneous or mediastinal. With longer term care, complications include tracheal irritation or infection.

More pressing aspects of tracheostomy tube care involve continuous patient monitoring, promoting a patent airway, and frequent hygienic care of the tube itself. The tube itself may leak, kink, may become dislodged, or even occlude with secretions or mucous

Clinical Small Animal Care: Promoting Patient Health through Preventative Nursing, First Edition. Kimm Wuestenberg.
© 2012 John Wiley & Sons, Inc. Published 2012 by John Wiley & Sons, Inc.

Table 14.1 Tracheostomy tube maintenance

Procedure	Frequency	Description	Supplies needed
Irrigation	Every 2-4 hours	Inject saline into tube, with or without coupage, use in conjunction to suctioning	2 mL saline (cats), 5-10 mL (dogs)
Suction preoxygenation	Immediately prior to suction	Connect Ambu bag to tube, administer four to five manual breaths using 100% oxygen	Oxygen source, electrocardiograph (ECG) monitor
Suction	Every 6-8 hours	Insert catheter until resistance noted, pulling back slightly, institute suction at −80 to −120 mmHg, twisting catheter as it is withdrawn Potential complications: hypoxia, lung collapse, cardiac arrhythmias, and hypotension	Sterile gloves, sterile red rubber catheter or other suitable suction tubing (less than 1/2 diameter of tracheostomy tube), Suction unit, with or without saline
Replace inner cannula	With suction procedure	Remove cannula, suction, then replace	A new or clean (sterile) cannula insert
Troubleshooting a dysfunctional tube	As needed	Remove inner cannula, deflate cuff, maneuver or manipulate tube placement, suction if possible, replace tube if needed, check oxygen source and connection when applicable, auscultate lungs and evaluate patient status	Oxygen, intubation equipment, new tracheostomy tube, pulse oximetry, ECG

plugs. Breath sounds should routinely be evaluated; the patient's tube requires irrigation every 2-4 hours and suctioning every 6-8 hours to promote pulmonary hygiene and a patent airway. Refer to Table 14.1 for procedure.

Tracheostomy tubes with inflatable cuffs should be inflated to a point where a slight leak can be heard on peak inspiration. Care should be taken to prevent overinflation, as this increased pressure can lead to tracheal tissue necrosis. Periodic deflation of the cuff does not necessarily prevent tracheal necrosis. Typically, tracheostomy tubes should be replaced once a week unless complications occur sooner (Table 14.1, Figs. 14.1-14.3).

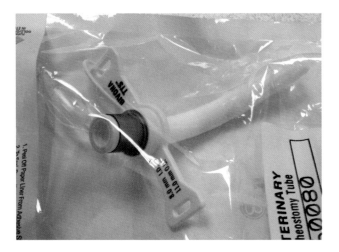

Figure 14.1 Packaged tracheostomy tube.

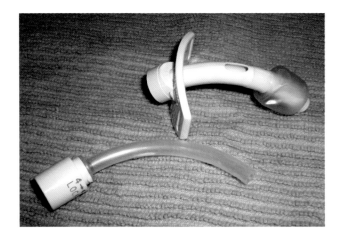

Figure 14.3 Tracheostomy tube and insert.

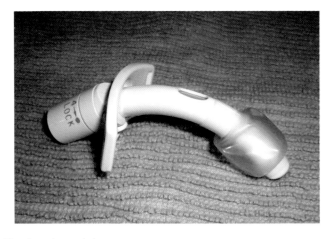

Figure 14.2 Tracheostomy tube.

Chapter references and further reading

K. Kinnerney (2009) Tracheostomy tube care. *Veterinary Technician the Complete Journal for the Veterinary Hospital Staff* **30**(2): 20-23.
D. Waldron (2003) Using tracheostomy tubes. Western Veterinary Conference.

Chapter 15
Chest Tube Care

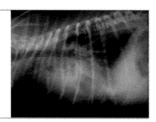

A thoracocentesis may be performed in patients suffering from a pneumothorax, pleural effusion, chylothorax, hemothorax, or pyothorax. Thoracocentesis may be used as a therapeutic or diagnostic purpose, sometimes serving both. As a general rule, once a thoracocentesis has been performed three times, a chest tube should be placed as the condition has not resolved. There are risks with performing a thoracocentesis, including an iatrogenic pneumothorax, puncture or laceration of a lung, or severe distress due to procedure restraint. Ensuring patient safety should always be a priority when performing a thoracocentesis. If the stress, anxiety, or resistance is too great, a reassessment is in order. Analgesics or sedatives may be required; patients may also benefit from oxygen therapy and medications, depending on the medical condition. For instance, a patient with heart failure and subsequent pleural effusion may benefit from a diuretic and oxygen therapy prior to attempting a thoracocentesis. However, in the instance of a pneumothorax, time is crucial, and a sedative or analgesic may ease the procedure. It is important to remember that patients in respiratory distress are very fragile and may succumb to procedure restraint. Patient mentation, mucous membrane color, and respiratory pattern and effort should be closely monitored.

Thoracostomy tubes are generally implemented when either effusion or air continuously builds, or postoperatively when a thoracotomy has been performed. There are commercially available chest tubes; however, red rubber catheters can also be used. The benefit of commercially available tubes is that most are made with a one-way valve, preventing air to enter the thoracic space. They often have multiple drainage holes as well, preventing occlusion of the catheter or tube.

With the initial placement of a chest tube, aspiration should be implemented every 15–30 minutes as volume and patient status permits, increasing aspiration as necessary to remove air or fluid. Intervals may gradually increase to 2–4 hours depending on fluid or air production and the patient status. Patients should be repositioned during aspiration, moving from lateral to sternal recumbency in the attempt to collect more fluid. When necessary, a continuous suction unit may be used. Some patients may produce a significant amount of fluid or air and never reach negative pressure with intermittent aspiration.

Clinical Small Animal Care: Promoting Patient Health through Preventative Nursing, First Edition.
Kimm Wuestenberg.

Chest tubes are placed between the seventh and ninth intercostals spaces and may be placed on either the left or right side. The skin over the 12th rib is manipulated cranially prior to insertion, leaving a subcutaneous tunnel between the entry into the thorax and the exit from the skin. This helps prevent infection and leakage of air and fluid, somewhat sealing the sites. Chest tubes should be kept covered with either a bandage or stockinet and handled in a sterile manner. The bandage material should be kept clean and dry and the tube clamped closed when not using a continuous suction drainage system. It is recommended to disinfect the chest tube every 8–12 hours, focusing on the distal end of the tube and seals or caps. The bandage should be stripped down and inspected at least once a day and the insertion site cleaned and observed for signs of infection. If signs of infection are present, the tube should be removed. If patient discomfort is noted, a local anesthetic may be injected through the tube to provide relief.

Cytological examination of aspirated contents should be performed every 24–48 hours. Sample analysis should include color, turbidity, and odor. Normal pleural fluid volume is less than 1mL/kg of body weight. It is typically clear to straw in color and may be clear to slightly turbid. Pleural fluid normally has no odor, few erythrocytes, a total protein less than 2.5–3 g/dL, and less than 10,000 nucleated cells per microliter, primarily neutrophils (75%). Exudates tend to be highly cellular with a high protein. Transudates have lower cell numbers with or without low protein levels. Septic samples will exhibit a marked increase in neutrophils, toxic neutrophils, and bacteria. Hemorrhage will be noted by the presence of blood and a peripheral packed cell volume (PCV) should be obtained and compared to the PCV of the chest fluid to rule out an active or recently active hemorrhage. A ruptured lymph duct may be noted by the presence of chyle and a total protein of 2–6 g/dL.

The patient with a chest tube should be monitored for signs of respiratory pattern changes, respiratory distress, and maintenance of normal vital sign parameters and level of consciousness. The tube should be kept clean, handled in an aseptic manner, and observed for signs of occlusion or leakage. The chest tube may become occluded with material or due to patient positioning. If a drainage system is used, proper troubleshooting of the system should be implemented on a regular basis or sooner if patient status begins to deteriorate. Fluid may leak around the tube insertion site so skin should be kept clean and a seal may be applied to help reduce leakage (such as an antibiotic ointment). The tube should remain covered and an Elizabethan collar placed when necessary. Chest tubes may become caught on kennel or cage doors, resulting in a pneumothorax if torn or uncapped. All caps, attachments, tubing, and additional instrumentation used should be secured. Once air or fluid production remains less than 2 mL/kg of body weight, or nonproductive for 12–24 hours, the drain may be removed. A light bandage is generally placed around the chest for 24 hours postremoval.

Chapter references and further reading

S. Erickson (2008) Thoracocentesis, chest tube management and arterial sampling. International Veterinary Emergency and Critical Care Symposium.

D. Schroeder, V. Skala, C. Nielsen (2005) Managing pyothorax in a dog. *Veterinary Technician the Complete Journal for the Veterinary Hospital Staff* **26**(5): 340–350.

Comprehensive Areas of Focus

Chapter 16

Cardiovascular Nursing

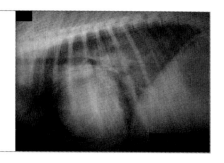

Basic anatomy and physiology overview

The heart is a muscle that holds the primary purpose of pumping blood to the tissues and organs of the body. The body's blood functions to deliver oxygen, nutrients, and hormones, among other necessities, to the body's tissues. The blood also carries away waste products from those tissues and it aids in the maintenance of the body's fluid balance. All tissues in the body need blood flow to deliver nutrients and carry away wastes. Cardiac preload (blood entering the heart) in conjunction with the rate and force of the heart pumping determines the cardiac output, or delivery of blood to the body tissues.

There are four chambers of the heart: the right and left atria (upper) and the right and left ventricles (lower). The atria are utilized as holding chambers while the ventricles of the heart perform the pumping or forward moving blood flow. There are four valves which open and close to direct the blood flow. The valves, in respect to blood flow, are the tricuspid valve, pulmonary valve, mitral valve, and aortic valve. Furthermore, the heart is surrounded by the pericardial sac, which holds a small amount of fluid to prevent friction as the heart pumps.

The cardiovascular system is divided into two divisions—pulmonary circulation and systemic circulation. As blood enters the right atrium via the vena cava, it travels through the tricuspid valve to the right ventricle and then to the pulmonary artery, which leads to the lungs. This cardiac blood flow is termed pulmonary circulation because the lungs are perfused by the right side of the heart. Once the gas exchange has occurred in the lungs, blood travels back to the heart via the pulmonary arteries and enters the left atrium, traveling through the mitral valve to the left ventricle, and finally out to the body via the aorta. Left-sided cardiac circulation is then termed systemic circulation (Fig. 16.1).

In order for the cardiovascular system to work efficiently, the valves and chambers must work efficiently and rhythmically. Adequate preload combined with effective cardiac contraction will determine the afterload, or perfusion to the body. If there is a

Clinical Small Animal Care: Promoting Patient Health through Preventative Nursing, First Edition. Kimm Wuestenberg.
© 2012 John Wiley & Sons, Inc. Published 2012 by John Wiley & Sons, Inc.

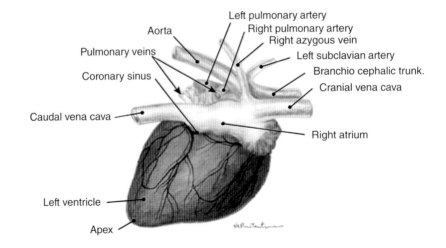

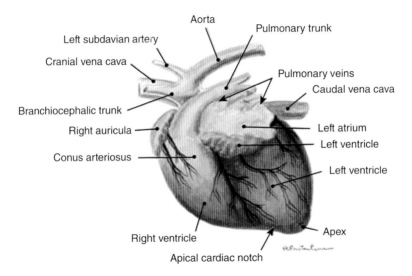

Figure 16.1 Diagram of the heart. Reprinted with permission from Akers, M. and Denbow, M. *Anatomy and Physiology of Domestic Animals*. Wiley-Blackwell, 2008.

decrease in blood flow, or if the cardiac pump itself is dysfunctional, the result is an inadequate outflow to the body (poor systemic circulation). The term systolic refers to the active phase (pumping) while diastolic refers to the relaxing or refilling phase of the cardiac cycle.

In addition to the anatomical makeup of the heart, the cardiac conduction system plays a role in performance. Each individual heart muscle cell has the ability to relax and contract spontaneously. Contraction (depolarization) occurs due to an electrical impulse across the cell membrane. Relaxation (repolarization) occurs as the membrane returns to resting state. Contraction and relaxation occurs via sodium, calcium, and potassium channels which alternately open and close, allowing the charged ions to flow across the membranes.

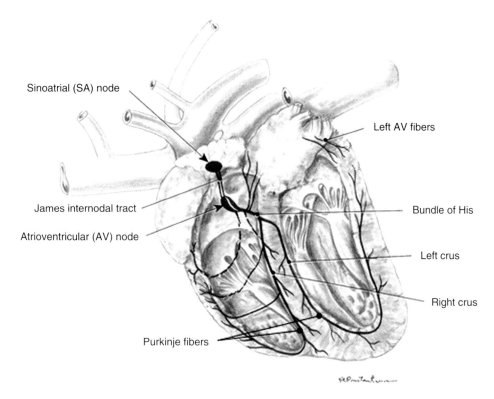

Figure 16.2 Conduction system of the heart. Reprinted with permission from Akers, M. and Denbow, M. *Anatomy and Physiology of Domestic Animals*. Wiley-Blackwell, 2008.

The cardiac conduction system is made up of the SA node, the AV node, the bundle of His, the right and left bundle branches, and the Purkinje fibers. The SA node (sino-atrial node) is the cardiac muscle located where the cranial vena cava meets the right atrium. The AV node (atrioventricular node) is in the septal wall of the right atrium. The bundle of His connects the AV node to the ventricular septum and separates into the right and left bundle branches. The bundle branches end at the Purkinje fibers, which are muscle fibers that are located beneath the endocardium. The SA node is the primary pacemaker of the heart by reason of conduction slowing as it travels further down the conduction system to the Purkinje fibers (Fig. 16.2).

Lastly, neuroendocrine influences play a role in cardiovascular system function. The sympathetic and parasympathetic systems can alter vessel dynamics (influencing blood pressure, thus delivery) as well as chronotropic and inotropic performance of the cardiac pump itself. If cardiac function and perfusion is impaired, neurohormonal responses ensue and inflammatory mediators contribute to a vicious cycle as decompensation occurs.

Assessing the cardiovascular patient

Considering the cardiovascular system has the capability to influence both the internal and external respiration of a patient, numerous scenarios could cascade in the cardiovascularly impaired patient. These are one of the more in-depth nursing cases in which detail to the patient is crucial and support staff is utilized to their full critical thinking potential. Any deviation from normal parameters or changes in patient status warrants investigation, if not already done.

Patients with cardiovascular conditions may display symptoms such as (but are not limited to) exercise intolerance, fatigue, cough which may or may not be productive, ascites, abdominal or labored breathing, and cyanosis. It's important to note that primary respiratory disease may present with similar symptoms as cardiovascular symptoms and differentiation between the two etiologies may be a challenging task.

Starting with the primary survey, patient mentation will allow for a quick triage of perfusion or cardiac output. As blood pressure decreases and impaired perfusion persists, the patient loses consciousness. Patient mental awareness gives a quick, short-term evaluation of hemodynamics as parameters may change acutely in the cardiac patient.

The assessment of cardiac function involves auscultation of the heart, monitoring pulses for quality and synchronicity as well as the color and capillary refill time (CRT) of the mucous membranes (MMs). It is important to note that with every heartbeat, a pulse should then follow. Some arrhythmias will cause a deviation in this normal pattern, thereby creating a situation where the heart may beat several times before a pulse is palpable, negatively affecting perfusion. Furthermore, it is important to appreciate that pale or cyanotic MM color is considered to be the last sign of internal hypoxia. There usually is a state of hypoperfusion which may be detected by assessing the cardiac output of the patient (heart rate, pulse quality and rhythm, blood pressure monitoring, etc.).

In the respiratory survey, attention to the respiratory rate, pattern, effort, and posture should be observed and documented in addition to any abnormal lung sounds auscultated. Along with respiratory difficulties, hyperthermia often occurs. It is important to consider monitoring the temperature of these patients and maintain euthermia through cooling techniques when indicated.

Common cardiovascular diseases and conditions

Pericardial disorders such as effusion and tamponade occur when the pericardial sac accumulates excessive fluid buildup. The cause may be due to pericarditis, which is an infection of the heart (fungal, bacterial, etc.) or tumor related (chemodectoma, hemangiosarcoma, etc.). A pericardial tamponade is a life-threatening effusion where the pressure from the excessive fluid around the heart is so great that the heart cannot function. This is an emergency situation requiring immediate attention. The fluid buildup prevents the cardiac muscle from performing, limiting cardiac output and tissue perfusion. These patients can progress to organ failure and death if the pressure is not relieved from the pericardial space.

Patients with pericardial effusion or tamponade may display signs similar to right-sided heart failure due to the decreased cardiac output. They may tire easily or appear weak. Upon auscultation, the heart may sound muffled, although heart sounds are often absent. Patient monitoring includes detail to mentation, blood pressure monitoring, and

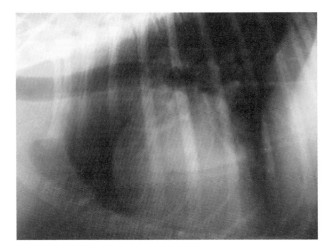

Figure 16.3 Pericardial effusion radiograph.

observing the respiratory pattern and effort for signs of dyspnea. An electrocardiogram will display electrical alternans and thoracic radiographs usually reveal a large, global heart. The patients' jugular veins may also be notably distended. Once the patient is stabilized, a pericardiocentesis should ensue, relieving the effusion. Surgical correction (pericardial window) may also be warranted in patients with a pericardial effusion or tamponade (Fig. 16.3).

Cardiomyopathies are a primary myocardial disease in which the function of the heart muscle deteriorates. Hypertrophic cardiomyopathy (HCM), dilative cardiomyopathy (DCM), and restrictive cardiomyopathy (RCM) fall into this category. In HCM (commonly seen in cats), the heart muscle thickens, making cardiac output a strenuous task for the heart. DCM is a condition in which the heart muscle has become dilated and enlarged, resulting in ineffective pumping action. DCM is seen in dogs and cats, but most often associated with large breed dogs. Cats can get DCM when their diet is taurine deficient. RCM is less common than HCM and DCM, but it is seen in cats. Fibrosis in the left ventricles causes dysfunction and they are unable to fill with blood, preventing adequate perfusion to the body.

Valvular disorders include stenosis (narrowing) and insufficiency (abnormal performance) of the heart valves. The most common valves associated with stenosis are the pulmonic and aortic valves (semilunar valves). Insufficient valves, also referred to as leaky valves, are most commonly associated with the AV valves (tricuspid and mitral valves).

Congenital disorders are defects in which the animal is born with and are not necessarily hereditary traits. These disorders can be divided into two sections—the failure of fetal structures to close and the failure of fetal structures to develop normally. Cardiac fetal structures which fail to close include atrial septal defects (ASDs) and patent ductus arteriosus (PDA). In an ASD, blood flows from the right atria to the left atria and vice versa, through a hole in the interatrial septum, causing a mix of venous and arterial blood. A PDA is a failure of the ductus arteriosus to close following birth. Blood continues to flow from the pulmonary artery directly into to the aorta, bypassing pulmonary circulation. Fetal structures which fail to develop normally include ventricular septal defect (VSD) and persistent right aortic arch (PRAA). A VSD involves the shunting of arterial and venous blood through a hole between the right and left ventricles in the ventricular septum. A PRAA occurs when the right arch of the aorta grows around the esophagus, causing a stricture. The fetal aorta is developed by a series of large vessels in which normally the left arch persists.

Congestive heart failure (CHF) is the end result of cardiac conditions such as fetal structure defects, heart muscle defects, valvular dysfunction, hypertension, endocarditis, and so on. When the failure occurs on the right side of the heart, the patient often develops ascites due to the inability of forward flow. Likewise, left-sided heart failure is often associated with pulmonary edema as blood traveling from the lungs to the left side of the heart is unable to circulate in an efficient manner. CHF affects the patients' kidney function due to poor perfusion as well as creating a situation where the patient is easily overexerted. It is important to keep in mind that many cardiac patients, not only CHF patients, can deteriorate rapidly and even succumb to the stresses of handling (Figs. 16.4 and 16.5).

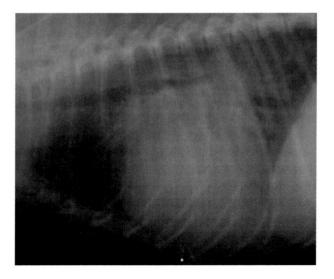

Figure 16.4 Radiograph of CHF and pulmonary edema in a dog.

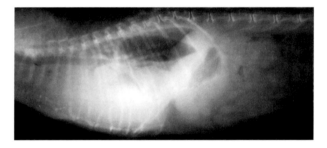

Figure 16.5 Radiograph of pleural effusion in a cat due to heart failure.

Patients with CHF often have secondary conditions such as pleural effusion, pulmonary edema, or ascites. These conditions can lead to dyspnea and usually require pharmaceutical intervention such as loop diuretics, positive inotropes, beta blockers, vasodilators, and so on depending on the cause of the CHF. Oxygen should be administered and if the patient has anxiety, sedatives may be warranted. Therapeutic thoracocentesis may be performed in the event of pleural effusion or significant ascites in which dyspnea is present. Relieving the fluid from the abdomen will allow the diaphragm to move further caudally, allowing more air into the lungs with inspirations.

Patient monitoring includes observing for signs of dyspnea, pale or cyanotic MMs, weak pulses and prolonged CRT, crackle sounds upon lung auscultation (pulmonary edema), and even hypothermia. In patients with pulmonary edema, white or pink frothy fluid may be noted from nostrils (fulminating pulmonary edema), or coughing of this fluid may occur.

Arrhythmias are a disorder of the rhythm, or synchronicity, of the heart beating. Arrhythmias are often classified as supraventricular (atrial) or ventricular, denoting the origination of the dysrythmia. In addition, bradyarrhythmias are associated with a slow heart rate (bradycardia), and tachyarrhythmias occur when there is a rapid heart rate (tachycardia). Considering that the electrical conductivity of the heart is associated with structure performance, a patient with an arrhythmia, whether primary or secondary, should be monitored as extensively as any other cardiovascularly impaired patient would.

A key nursing skill for detecting arrhythmias is to always palpate pulses while auscultating the heart. For every heartbeat, a pulse should then follow. Often pulses are obtained, or heart rates are obtained but they are not performed together, which is essential in detecting certain types of arrhythmias. A patient with a heart rate of 142 beats per minute (bpm) may display a pulse rate of 116 bpm. Arrhythmias are often overlooked as support staff may obtain one vital sign without the other. The heart should also be auscultated as rhythm and rate can be an indicator of arrhythmias (Fig. 16.6).

Hemodynamics refers to the circulation of blood flow. The force of blood against the walls of vessels as it moves is termed blood pressure. A specific pressure must be met to ensure that tissues and vital organs are perfused in the body. Hypertension is a condition in which blood pressure is above, or higher, than normal range. Causes can be primary or secondary such as in renal disease, pheochromocytoma, lead toxicity, and so on. Hypotension is then a condition in which blood pressure falls below the normal range. It may be due to (but not limited to) impaired states such as anesthesia or shock. In both scenarios, blood pressure monitoring is a key tool. A hypertensive patient may suffer from epistaxis, hematuria, and ocular hemorrhage due to the excessive forcing of blood. Mydriasis may be noted and acute blindness due to retinal detachment can occur. The hypotensive patient may progress to a critical shock status.

Shock is considered to be an imbalance between delivered oxygen and consumed oxygen where the former is deficient. During the initial stages of shock, cellular hypoxia causes an energy deficit as mitochrondia are no longer able to generate adenosine triphosphate (ATP). Anaerobic metabolism ensues, causing the pH to fall, leading to metabolic acidosis. An acute compensatory sympathetic response causes major arteries and veins to constrict. Initially, capillaries constrict, causing a decreased perfusion to

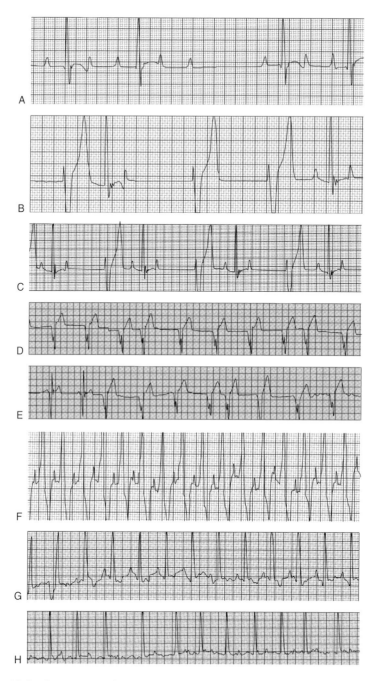

Figure 16.6 Common cardiac arrhythmias. A. Second-degree atrioventricular (AV) block. Note the third recorded impulse is missing a QRS complex following the P wave. B. Ventricular premature complexes (VPCs). The first, third, and fourth complexes are all VPCs (uniform/unifocal). C. Bigeminy. Normal complexes alternating with VPCs. D. Sustained VPCs. There are no normal complexes seen. E. Multiform (multifocal) VPCs. The first two complexes are normal, while the rest are VPCs. F. Bundle branch block. This appears similar to ventricular tachycardia (VTach) but P waves are present. G. Atrial premature complexes. Note lack of baseline; the T wave immediately proceeds into P waves. H. Atrial fibrillation in a 13-year-old German Shepherd dog. Note the "shaky" baseline with no definitive P waves.

tissues; however, as anaerobic metabolism progresses, blood flow into the capillaries is increased as outflow is restricted, causing a volume shift of blood accumulating in the venules. This local "pooling" is responsible for the misdistribution of blood flow. Fluid and protein then leaks into the surrounding tissues, which concentrates the blood and increases viscosity on a microvascular level. Prolonged vasoconstriction results in loss of blood flow to vital organs which were previously protected by arterial shunting. The end result is catastrophic as this terminal phase of shock is reached.

Other cardiovascular conditions commonly seen are distal aortic thromboembolism and caval syndrome. Patients with aortic thromboembolism (ATE, "saddle thrombus") are usually feline and may or may not have a documented history of cardiomyopathy. ATE occurs when a thrombus from the left atrium is released into circulation and occludes the flow to peripheral arteries. These patients usually present with an acute episode of hind-end paralysis or paresis and lack pulses. Hind extremities are more often affected, but forelimbs can be affected as well. These patients are usually in pain, may be vocal, and sometimes will present with respiratory distress (possibly due to pulmonary thromboembolism).

Patient nursing care of the ATE patient includes pain management, oxygen administration if needed, physical therapy, and supportive care. The administration of thrombolytic agents may influence nursing implications as these medications come with a wide variety of potential complications which can make for a challenging case. In extreme cases, the patient may undergo surgery to remove the thrombus, or amputation of a limb which has suffered necrosis.

Caval syndrome occurs when adult heartworms (*Dirofilaria immitis*) occlude the tricuspid valve and cause right-sided heart failure due to the presence of worms in both the right atria and ventricle. These patients are generally weak and have pale MMs with a prolonged CRT due to reduced cardiac output. The jugular veins may also be distended and the patient may be tachypneic (Tables 16.1 and 16.2).

Table 16.1   Patient care quick reference guide

Parameter	Evaluation and diagnostics	Potential interventions
Mentation: dulled, obtunded, stuperous, comatose or unconscious	Check response to stimuli, heart rate, pulse quality, obtain blood pressure or central venous pressure (CVP), oxygen saturation, and monitor urine output	Oxygen administration (hypoxia), colloid administration and pharmaceutical intervention (hypotension), urinary catheter placement
Heart: new murmur, new arrhythmia, bradycardia or tachycardia	Check pulse quality and synchronicity, perform diagnostic ECG, balance fluid ins/outs (murmur)	Pharmaceutical intervention, continuous ECG monitoring, adjust fluid therapy, and further diagnostics if warranted
		(Continued)

Table 16.1 (*continued*)

Parameter	Evaluation and diagnostics	Potential interventions
Perfusion: hyperdynamic, bounding, strong pulse quality; poor, weak or thread pulse quality; pulse deficits; prolonged CRT; muddy, pale or cyanotic MM	Check mentation, auscultate heart, obtain blood pressure, oxygen saturation, diagnostic ECG, consider CVP or arterial blood pressure (ABP) if available	Oxygen administration, colloid administration (hypotension), pharmaceutical intervention, continuous multiparameter monitoring; therapeutic pericardiocentesis if warranted
Respiratory pattern: inspiratory or expiratory dyspnea, bradypnea, tachypnea, orthopnea, abdominal or labored respirations	Auscultate lungs bilaterally, check oxygen saturation, patient may require minimal handling to prevent respiratory arrest	Oxygen administration, pharmaceutical intervention, therapeutic thoracocentesis or abdominocentesis if warranted
Hyperthermia: due to dyspnea-induced anxiety	Check oxygen chamber temperature, confirm oxygen delivery to patient, evaluate fluid therapy temperature and discontinue the use of warmed IV fluids	Consider alternative oxygen delivery routes, apply ice packs to oxygen chamber, direct a circulating fan towards patient if possible, offer water to patient if possible

Table 16.2 Cardiac auscultation points

Anatomic evaluation	Stethoscope location (canine)	Stethoscope location (feline)
Tricuspid valve	Low right, third to fourth intercostal space	Right, fourth to fifth at costochondral junction
Pulmonary valve	Low left, third intercostal space	Left, second to third intercostal space
Mitral valve	Left, fifth at costochondral junction	Left, fifth to sixth costochondral junction
Aortic valve	High left, fourth intercostal space	Left, second to third above the pulmonic region

Chapter references and further reading

B. Brewer (2003) Echocardiography basics: echocardiographic findings in acquired heart disease. *Veterinary Technician the Complete Journal for the Veterinary Hospital Staff* **24**(11): 781-789.

A. Campbell (2008) Pericardial effusion. International Veterinary Emergency and Critical Care Symposium.

K. Glaze (1998a) Congenital heart disease: part I. *Veterinary Technician the Complete Journal for the Veterinary Hospital Staff* **19**(3): 169-179.

K. Glaze (1998b) Congenital heart disease: part II. *Veterinary Technician the Complete Journal for the Veterinary Hospital Staff* **19**(5): 339-347.

A. Gottlieb (2004) Compassion for a cat with saddle thrombus. *Veterinary Technician the Complete Journal for the Veterinary Hospital Staff* **25**(6): 430-432.

P. Plummer (2009) Caval syndrome and pulmonary arterial hypertension. *Veterinary Technician the Complete Journal for the Veterinary Hospital Staff* **30**(6): 16-21.

J. Romich (1998) You've gotta have heart. *Veterinary Technician the Complete Journal for the Veterinary Hospital Staff* **19**(5): 331-336.

J. Rush (2008) Heart failure in dogs and cats. International Veterinary Emergency and Critical Care Symposium.

R. Stepien (2003) Interpreting heart murmurs. Western Veterinary Conference.

L. Waddell (2008) Monitoring the cardiovascular compromised patient. International Veterinary Emergency and Critical Care Symposium.

S. Ware (2001) Facilitating the management of heart failure patients. Wild West Veterinary Conference.

Chapter 17
Regard for the Respiratory Patient

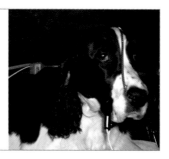

The respiratory system overview

The respiratory system consists of the lungs and air passageways which lead to the lungs. Several structures exist to modify the air en route to the alveoli of the lungs, filtering, warming, and moistening it. The respiratory system is also involved in vocalizing.

The upper respiratory tract consists of the nose, the paranasal sinuses, pharynx, larynx, and trachea. The external nose is comprised of the nasal planum, nares, and philtrum, while the internal nose is made up of the nasal septum and chonchae, or turbinates. The paranasal sinuses are bilateral, symmetrical openings of the skull. The pharynx is a passageway that connects the oral cavity to the esophagus and the nasal passage with the larynx. There are three divisions of the pharynx: the nasopharynx, oropharynx, and laryngopharynx. The nasopharynx is the respiratory portion of the division. It extends from the caudal aspect of the internal nares, contains the hard palate, and terminates at the laryngopharynx. The oropharynx is a continuation of the oral cavity and contains the soft palate, also terminating at the laryngopharynx. The larynx contains the epiglottis, cartilages (thyroid, arytenoids, and cricoid), ventricular, and vocal folds. The pharynx continues to the esophagus and the larynx continues to the trachea. The trachea directs inhaled air from the upper airway to the lungs. It divides into two portions at an area called the tracheal bifurcation, leading to the left and right mainstem bronchi (Fig. 17.1).

The lower respiratory tract is housed in the thorax and contains the tracheal bifurcation and the lungs. The mainstem bronchi divide into smaller bronchi, which subdivide further into the smallest air passageways called bronchioles. Gas exchange occurs in the alveoli residing at the terminal end of these bronchioles. The caudal border of the thorax is formed by a dome-shaped musculotendinous structure called the diaphragm. The parietal pleura lines the ribs and musculature of the thorax while the visceral pleura

Clinical Small Animal Care: Promoting Patient Health through Preventative Nursing, First Edition. Kimm Wuestenberg.
© 2012 John Wiley & Sons, Inc. Published 2012 by John Wiley & Sons, Inc.

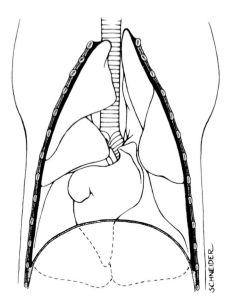

Figure 17.1 Ventral view of the thoracic cavity: lungs, trachea, and diaphragm. Reprinted with permission from Adams, D. *Canine Anatomy: A Systemic Study, Fourth Edition.* Blackwell Publishing, 2004.

lines the lungs. A vacuum exists between the parietal and visceral pleuras, keeping the lungs inflated. If this vacuum is lost, the lungs will be unable to inflate, resulting in respiratory distress (pneumothorax). Dogs and cats have four right lung lobes (cranial, middle, caudal, and accessory) and two left lung lobes (cranial and caudal). The cranial left lung lobe has a cranial and caudal portion.

Respiratory physiology involves ventilation and respiration. Inspiratory ventilation is air movement into the lungs, while expiratory ventilation is moving the air out of the lungs. Inspiratory ventilation is largely attributed to the action of the diaphragm and the external intercostal muscles. The lungs move with the thoracic wall due to the vacuum, and as the wall expands, the lungs also expand, allowing an influx of air. Expiratory ventilation is attributed to abdominal and intercostal muscle action, forcing the diaphragm cranially (Table 17.1).

There is a volume of air in the respiratory tract, which is nonfunctional in gas exchange, called "dead space." Anatomical dead space consists of the conducting airways—nasal passages, trachea, bronchi, and bronchioles. Physiological dead space is the volume of the lung that does not eliminate carbon dioxide. In healthy animals, this volume is nearly zero but disease states can result in an increase in physiological dead space.

Respiration is the gas exchange between oxygen and carbon dioxide. Internal respiration occurs on a cellular level in the capillaries of the body's tissues while external respiration occurs in the alveoli of the lungs. Oxygen passes through the alveolar walls via diffusion and red blood cells remove the oxygen and carry it to the body tissues (Fig. 17.2).

Table 17.1 Lung volumes

Total lung capacity	Maximum volume of air the lungs can hold
Vital capacity	Maximum volume of air that can be inspired and expired
Tidal volume	Volume of air that is inspired and expired during normal breathing
Functional residual capacity	The volume of air present in the lungs following maximum expiration It is determined by the sum of residual volume and expiratory reserve volume

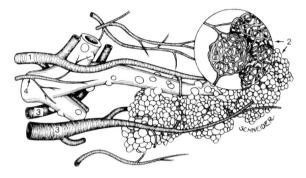

Figure 17.2 The terminal branch of the airway including alveoli and vasculature. Reprinted with permission from Adams, D. *Canine Anatomy: A Systemic Study, Fourth Edition.* Blackwell Publishing, 2004.

Ventilation is involuntary, regulated by a central controller located in the brain and peripheral controllers in the lungs, thorax, and carotid bodies. The medulla is responsible for the rate of respirations. Low carbon dioxide levels in blood decrease the rate of respirations while an increased carbon dioxide level in the blood increases the rate of respiration. Oxygen content of blood does not control respiratory rate. Chemoreceptors respond to the amount of carbon dioxide detected in blood. There are receptors in the lung which limit the expansion of lung lobes and respond to irritants (i.e., cough reflex). Upper airway receptors function in the sneeze and cough reflex.

Upper respiratory conditions may be accompanied by a stridor (audible sound created on inspiration) or stertor (expiratory sound). In upper respiratory conditions, an inspiratory dyspnea may also be noted. Nasopharyngeal conditions include brachycephalic syndrome, epistaxis, rhinitis, and sinusitis. Neoplastic tumors may also occur at the mucosa of the nasal passages. The most commonly seen are nasal adenocarcinoma and SCC (squamous cell carcinoma). Brachycephalic syndrome occurs in short-nosed breeds such as pugs, bulldogs, Pekingese, Persian cats, and so on. Brachycephalic breeds tend to have stenotic nares (narrow nasal passageways), an elongated soft palate which may obstruct the larynx, everted laryngeal saccules (the space between the vocal folds and the arytenoids cartilages pouches out into the glottis), and a hypoplastic trachea where the trachea is smaller in proportion to the dog's size. Each of these can lead to respiratory difficulties, particularly in episodes of stress or anxiety. It is important to recognize that these breeds can easily become overheated, either in the environment or upon

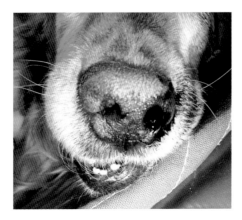

Figure 17.3 Patient with epistaxis.

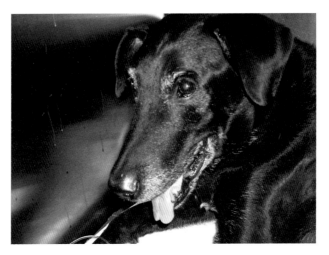

Figure 17.4 Using a white towel or blanket can help monitor the bleeding.

clinical handling. Muzzles should be used with extreme caution in the brachycephalic breeds.

Epistaxis, or nosebleed, can have many causes; trauma, foreign bodies (foxtail, blade of grass), coagulopathies (thrombocytopenia), neoplasia, and *Ehrlichia* (tick fever) are some common causes. Treatment usually involves maintaining hemostasis in cases of severe bleeding. Epinephrine, which is a vasoconstrictor, can be administered intranasally, with or without using gauze packing or umbilical tape. Sedation may be helpful, and less movement will usually result in less irritation and dislodging of the clot (Figs. 17.3 and 17.4).

Rhinitis is an infection or inflammation of the nasal passages. It can be bacterial, viral, fungal, or parasitic. Bacterial is usually secondary to a foreign body, or an oronasal fistula resulting from an infected tooth root. Viral causes include the upper airway disease complexes such as distemper, parainfluenza, adenovirus type 2 in the dog, and rhinotracheitis, calici, and chlamydia in the cat. Fungal infections are seen most often in the dolichocephalic breeds (long nose). The fungal spores colonize in the turbinates and grow, destroying the turbinate bones. The fungus is usually *Coccidioides*, *Aspergillus* or *Cryptococcus*. Lastly, parasitic infections can lead to rhinitis. *Pneumonyssoides caninum* is a mite that can infect the dog's nasal and sinus passages. It is often an overlooked cause of chronic sneezing and epistaxis in the dog. Sinusitis is an infection or inflammation of the sinus cavities. It often accompanies rhinitis and can also be bacterial, fungal, viral, parasitic, or allergic.

The pharynx is mostly skeletal muscle. The two most commonly seen problems concerning the pharynx include paralysis and pharyngitis. Patients with pharyngeal paralysis may have difficulty swallowing and may aspirate stomach contents, leading to aspiration pneumonia. Pharyngitis occurs when there is inflammation or infection of the pharynx. Common conditions affecting the larynx include laryngeal spasm, stenosis, collapse, and laryngitis, which is an inflammation or infection of the larynx. Laryngeal spasm occurs when the cartilages of the trachea spasm and cause obstruction of the airway. Cats are particularly prone to this condition, especially when endotracheal intubation is attempted. It can be avoided by using a careful, gentle intubation technique as well as topically applying a local anesthetic such as lidocaine. Laryngeal stenosis occurs when the larynx scars and becomes unable to open completely. Laryngeal collapse or paralysis ("Lar-Par") is a medical emergency if the animal is unable to adequately move air. The laryngeal cartilages are unable to move out of the glottis and subsequent airway obstruction occurs. Usually, the animal will be sedated and intubated to establish a patent airway. Once respirations normalize, the animal may be extubated and kept mildly sedated. Surgical correction may be required and is often recommended.

Tracheal conditions include tracheitis, tracheal stenosis (narrowing), and tracheal collapse. Tracheitis occurs from an infection or inflammation of the trachea. Tracheal stenosis can occur following trauma or infection or it may be hereditary. With trauma or infection, the trachea may become scarred, leading to stenosis. Depending on the severity, surgical correction may be required. Tracheal collapse is commonly seen in toy breeds such as the Yorkshire terrier. Tracheal collapse causes upper airway obstruction resulting in dyspnea, stress, and anxiety. These patients often display a classic "goose honk" sound as they attempt to move air. Initial treatment usually involves sedation and intubation in severe cases. Surgical correction may follow, where tracheal rings are placed as a stent to open the trachea (Fig. 17.5).

Nursing observations of patients with upper airway disease consist of monitoring respiratory rate, effort, and patterns. Orthopneic breathing, where a patient postures with neck extension, is a clear sign of dyspnea. The patient is trying to open the airways by extending the neck. In addition to observing respiratory patterns and effort, mentation should be continuously assessed. The change in breathing pattern and effort will be an initial indicator of dyspnea; however, if these signs are not detected, the patient's mentation will dull as hypoxia ensues. It is imperative to prevent this by clinically monitoring the respiratory patient at all times. Any animal with the respiratory compromised should be placed in a location where continuous monitoring can take place.

Rapid respirations should be evaluated to determine if the patient is dyspneic and tachypneic or nervous, anxious, or painful. Any time a patient is unable to exchange

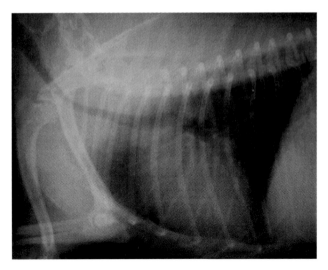

Figure 17.5 Lateral radiograph of tracheal stenosis in a Yorkshire terrier.

air, hyperthermia is a true risk. Temperatures should be frequently evaluated with modifications in the environment to maintain euthermia. Circulating air fans can be used, as well as placing ice packs in the kennel or allowing the pet to rest on a cool, damp towel. If thermoregulation is not achieved, it is possible that further measures may need to be taken. It may be necessary to sedate and intubate an anxious, hyperthermic pet to control breathing and thermoregulate. Additionally, if upper airway dyspnea persists, a tracheotomy may be indicated to allow adequate ventilation. Oxygen therapy may or may not benefit the patient with upper airway disease, depending on the nature or location of the problem. For instance, if a patient has laryngeal paralysis, placing a nasal oxygen cannula will not benefit the patient as the obstruction occurs past the point of oxygen delivery. Pulse oximetry or blood gas analysis can be beneficial to monitor in patients with upper airway disease.

Lower respiratory diseases include those of the thorax, the lung parenchyma, and the diaphragm. Thoracic conditions commonly seen are pneumothorax, pleural effusion, and pleuritis (Fig. 17.6).

Pneumothorax occurs when there is air in the pleural space. This is usually due to trauma, but a "spontaneous" pneumothorax can occur when diseased lung tissue ruptures (bulla) and enters the pleural space via the lungs. A tension pneumothorax or closed pneumothorax occurs when air enters the pleural space and is unable to exit. This is the most deadly type of pneumothorax. The patient becomes "barrel chested" and death ensues due to severe lung collapse. An open pneumothorax occurs when there is an opening in the thoracic wall, providing air movement into and out of the pleural space. Lung tissue may be exposed in an open pneumothorax. When air enters into the pleural space during a pneumothorax, the natural vacuum is decreased or no longer exists. Immediate treatment for pneumothorax involves thoracocentesis or chest tube placement. In cases of an open pneumothorax, plastic wrap can be used to bandage the opening and a thoracocentesis is performed (Fig. 17.6, Table 17.2).

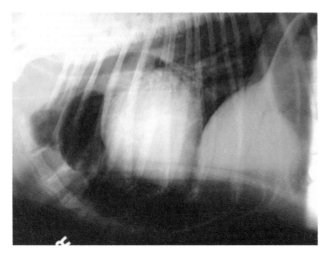

Figure 17.6 Lateral radiograph of a pneumothorax; note the "floating" heart.

Table 17.2 Clinical recognition of pneumothorax and pleural effusions

Clinical recognition of pneumothorax	Clinical recognition of pleural effusion
• Shallow, rapid respirations (tachypnea)	• Respiratory effort
• Dyspneic, open-mouth breathing	• Distended chest
• Diminished heart and lung sounds	• With or without cyanosis, pallor
• With or without "barrel chest" (tension pneumothorax)	• Quiet lung sounds *ventrally*
• With or without lung tissue exposure (open pneumothorax)	• Loud breath sounds *dorsally*
• Can be "spontaneous" but usually have a history of trauma	• With or without murmur, history of heart disease or trauma
	• With or without ascites
	• With or without jugular distension

A flail chest presents when two or more fractures occur on three or more ribs, causing instability. The affected area of the chest moves in during inspiration and out during expiration, which is the opposite of what normally occurs. This condition is usually seen as a result of vehicular trauma or bite wounds, especially when a larger animal has attacked a smaller one in the thoracic region. External support can be implemented by bandaging the chest or suturing tongue depressors to the site, stabilizing the fracture. Surgery is typically performed 24 hours later unless the condition worsens. The patient is to be placed flail side down until surgical correction is performed (Fig. 17.7).

Pleural effusion occurs when there is fluid buildup in the pleural space. This fluid can be transudative, exudative, or can be of another type (i.e., chylous). Pleuritis, or inflammation of the pleura, creates a friction sound upon lung auscultation. Pleuritis causes

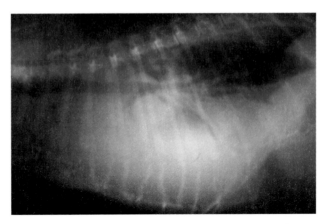

Figure 17.7 Lateral radiograph of a pleural effusion; note the classing "leafing" of the lung.

a large amount of fluid production and subsequent respiratory impairment. In chronic cases, a pleurodesis may be performed to minimize fluid production.

Bronchitis or bronchiolitis is an infection or inflammation of the bronchi. It can be viral, bacterial, or allergic in origin and is a fairly common problem in the dog and cat. Most cases start out as allergic and then a secondary bacterial infection occurs. Bronchitis causes excess mucous production and a productive cough. Over time, the small airways become thickened and the animal has decreased vital capacity.

Chronic obstructive pulmonary disease (COPD) is when chronic inflammation of the lung tissue results in fibrosis (scarring) of the lung tissue. This makes inspiration and expiration difficult, resulting in poor gas exchange.

Emphysema is often a result of chronic scarring (fibrosis) of the lung tissue. The lungs lose the ability to exhale efficiently, resulting in an increased abdominal effort upon expiration. Asthma or allergic bronchospasm is a common problem in the cat. Wheezing will be noted, along with a mixed inspiratory/expiratory dyspnea.

Pneumonia is an infection of the lungs and can be bacterial, fungal, or viral. The alveolus becomes flooded with liquid and cellular debris such as white blood cells or bacteria. Animals with pneumonia will have a productive cough. Some causes of pneumonia include (but are not limited to) atelectasis, near drowning, and aspiration pneumonia. Pneumonia can lead to pulmonary edema; however, there are many causes of pulmonary edema and it can be difficult to distinguish the two. Acute respiratory distress syndrome (ARDS) is a severe form of pulmonary edema. It results from trauma, shock, sepsis, or some other insult to the lung which alters the permeability of the alveolar cells. Unfortunately, ARDS is associated with a high mortality rate (Table 17.3).

Thrombosis may occur in the lungs with some cardiac conditions as well as inflammatory conditions. Pulmonary thromboembolism (PTE) is when a blood clot in the lung prevents a portion of the lung tissue from receiving blood, resulting in respiratory distress and hypoxia. Severe thrombosis can ultimately lead to death. Aortic thromboembolism (ATE or "saddle thrombus") occurs when a blood clot becomes lodged in the distal aorta and may accompany a PTE in some cases (Table 17.4).

Table 17.3 Causes of pulmonary edema

Causes of pulmonary edema	Mechanism
Congestive heart failure (CHF)	Inadequate cardiac function leading to altered blood flow
Electrocution	The electrical shock alters the permeability of the cells
Smoke inhalation	Smoke damages the cells, altering permeability
Heat stroke	Change in temperature alters permeability
Anaphylaxis (cats)	The lungs are the shock organ for cats
Iatrogenic	Fluid overload by veterinary personnel

Table 17.4 Examples of ventilation-perfusion mismatch

Ventilation-perfusion mismatch (V/Q mismatch)	Example
The lung is ventilated but not perfused (oxygen present, but no blood delivery)	Pulmonary thromboembolism
The lung is perfused but not ventilated (blood delivery, but no oxygen)	Pneumothorax

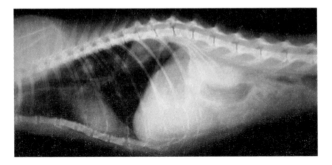

Figure 17.8 Lateral radiographs of lung metastasis in a feline, Tommy.

The lung is also a common site for metastatic disease; however, lung neoplasia may be primary. Cancers involving the thorax may affect the respiratory system of a patient due to pleural effusion, lung consolidation, or the tumor size or location (Fig. 17.8).

Nursing implications of lower respiratory disease are similar to those of the upper airway. Like upper airway disease, these patients will display orthopneic breathing, increased respiratory effort, changes in pattern as dyspnea progresses, and loss of mentation. Unlike many upper airway diseases, nasal oxygen cannulas may be beneficial to the patient. Additionally, therapeutic thoracocentesis (or abdominocentesis in cases of ascites) may be palliative and potentially curative in cases such as pneumothorax (Fig. 17.9).

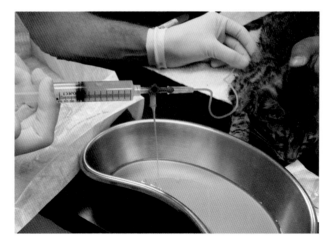

Figure 17.9 Palliative thoracocentesis in an 8-month-old kitten diagnosed with FIP at 2 months of age.

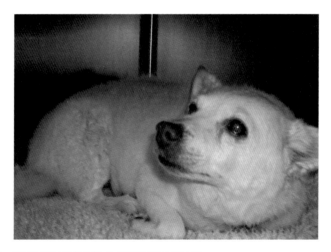

Figure 17.10 Neck extension in a dyspneic patient.

Nursing observations and interventions of the patient suffering from respiratory disease are an essential and potentially life-saving aspect of clinical care. The nursing staff should anticipate intense monitoring, evaluating, and critical thinking of stages to follow in the disease process.

Respiratory patients should be kept in an area where they are in constant supervision and an oxygen source is close. Adequate ventilation should be frequently (if not continuously) assessed. The patients' respiratory pattern, rate, and effort should always be assessed along with frequent auscultation of lung sounds. Inadequate ventilation can also lead to patient stress, thus exacerbating dyspnea. Respiratory patterns should be visually assessed and audibly evaluated prior to handling to prevent an episode of stress-induced respiratory arrest. It should be recognized that cyanosis is one of the last stages of dyspnea and the respiratory pattern changes are one of the first signs (Figs. 17.10 and 17.11).

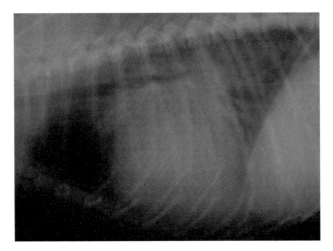

Figure 17.11 Lateral radiographs of patient in Fig. 17.10; cardiomegaly and pulmonary edema.

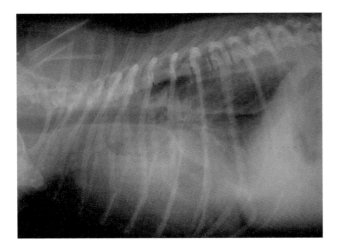

Figure 17.12 Lateral radiograph of pleural effusion due to lymphoma.

Patients who suffer from pleural effusions tend to have decreased heart and lung sounds upon auscultation. A variety of rales can be heard with airways diseases. Traumatic injury to the respiratory system should be considered a life-threatening emergency requiring immediate care. Thoracic trauma can result in pneumothorax, hemothorax, flail chest, and more. Keep in mind that nonthoracic traumas such as tracheal injury, snake envenomation, head trauma, or foreign bodies can also result in respiratory distress (Figs. 17.12–17.14).

Fluid therapy in respiratory patients requires a constant assessment in efforts to prevent overload. Some patients require fluid therapy to aid in tissue perfusion; however, an overload of fluid therapy may contribute to pulmonary dysfunction. The patient

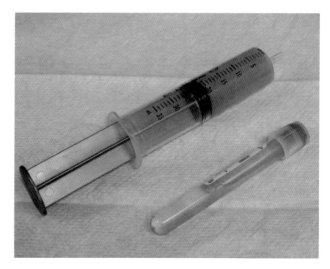

Figure 17.13 Fluid removed by thoracocentesis.

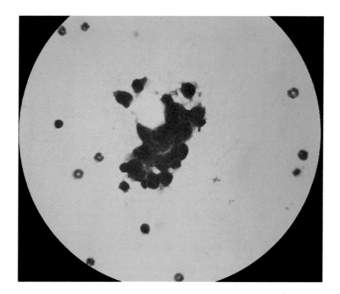

Figure 17.14 Microscopic examination of sample.

should be assessed by skin turgor, balancing fluid input and output, and utilizing laboratory tests such as packed cell volume/total solids (PCV/TS) and electrolytes.

Nebulization and chest physiotherapy may be indicated in some respiratory conditions such as pneumonia. If the patients' status allows, slow, short walks will help clear
the airways of secretions as exercise promotes this natural process.

The first priority in a patient suffering from respiratory distress is administering
oxygen and ensuring that a patent airway and ventilation has been established. Some
patients suffering from respiratory distress require sedation or anesthesia, endotracheal intubation, and manual ventilation to stabilize.

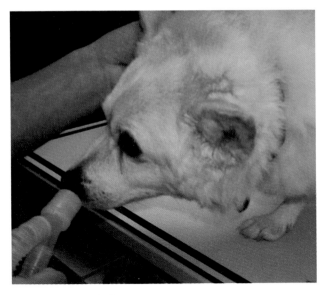

Figure 17.15 Administration of "flow-by" oxygen.

Oxygen delivery techniques

Oxygen can be delivered to the dyspneic patient in several ways. The main consider-ations when delivering oxygen should be effectiveness and patient stress level. The dyspneic patient is a high-risk patient and care should be taken to ensure comfort and subsequent easing of respirations (Fig. 17.15).

Oxygen kennels and chambers are available for delivering oxygen. The downfall of this method of delivery is that it restricts the technician from physically monitoring the patient. As the kennel or chamber door opens, oxygen is released from the kennel and the patient is no longer receiving high oxygen content. These kennels and chambers can also get warm, contributing to panting and in return furthering dyspnea. They oftentimes take several minutes to fill to an acceptable level of oxygen.

Oxygen masks and Elizabethan collars (E-collars) may be used to deliver oxygen. This allows for hands-on patient monitoring of the veterinary staff. Some patients undergo stress while wearing the E-collar or having the mask in close proximity, so again, care should be taken to recognize discomfort and stress levels. These devices must also have a means for the patients' carbon dioxide to be removed. An opening in the E-collar and removing the rubber seal of a face mask will ensure the patient's exhaled carbon dioxide is released from the devices and the patient will not be rebreathing the carbon dioxide (Fig. 17.16). Alternatively, a "flow-by" technique may be used, delivering oxygen without the use of a mask.

Nasal oxygen cannulas and catheters allow for hands-on patient nursing and are often well tolerated by the dyspneic patient. The catheter is inserted into the nostril and placed to the medial canthus using a lubricant, a topical anesthetic agent, and suture (or staples). The oxygen tubing is then connected to the nasal catheter. Human oxygen

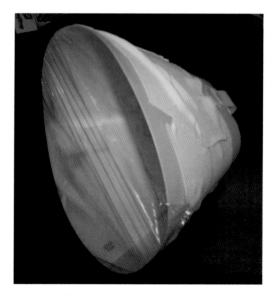

Figure 17.16 An E-collar modified with plastic wrap to create an oxygen collar; note the opening to ensure CO_2 outlet.

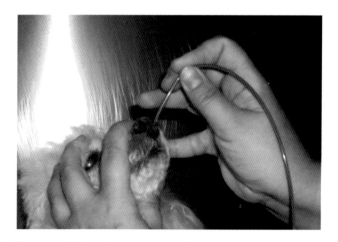

Figure 17.17 Placement of nasal oxygen cannula.

cannulas may be used, but stabilizing the placement may prove to be challenging (Fig. 17.17).

Lastly, a tracheal catheter or tracheostomy tube may be placed in the event of upper airway obstruction (laryngeal paralysis, tumors, foreign body obstruction, etc.). If the upper airway is not obstructed and the patient is severely dyspneic, sedation and endotracheal tube placement with manual (or ventilator) respirations may be beneficial to the patient (tracheal collapse, tracheal edema, pulmonary edema, etc.; Table 17.5).

Table 17.5 Lung auscultation reference and breath sounds

Lung auscultation reference	
Four quadrant	Craniodorsal; caudodorsal; cranioventral; and caudoventral
	Left and right side evaluation
Breath sounds	
Normal	
Vesicular	Lung parenchyma; best heard on inspiration
Bronchial	Trachea and large bronchi; best heard on expiration
Adventitious	Dry or moist rales; note location (i.e., tracheal vs. pleural)
Crackles	Fluid, mucus, or thicken walls of small airways
	Dry crackles : Solid material in bronchi or trachea
	Moist crackles: air movement through fluid
	Crepitant: fine crackles
Rhonchus	Dry, coarse rale in bronchial tubes
Grunt	Quick, sharp sound made when air is forced against (closed) glottis
Friction	Abrasive sound synchronous with respiration; caused by inflammation of serous surfaces in pleural cavity (i.e., pleuritis)
Wheezes	High-pitched sound, usually upon expiration (i.e., bronchitis)
Dull/muffled	Collapse or consolidation (i.e., pneumothorax, hydrothorax)
Peristaltic	Sounds made by gastrointestinal (GI) tract (i.e., diaphragmatic hernia)

Chapter references and further reading

A. Breton (2009) Acute lung injury and acute respiratory distress syndrome. *Veterinary Technician the Complete Journal for the Veterinary Hospital Staff* **30**(10): 26-30.

C. Hedlund (2003a) Brachycephalic syndrome. Western Veterinary Conference.

C. Hedlund (2003b) Evaluation of laryngeal disease. Western Veterinary Conference.

C. Hedlund (2003c) Laryngeal paralysis. Western Veterinary Conference.

C. Hedlund (2003d) Tracheal collapse. Western Veterinary Conference.

B. Marcucci (2004a) Feline asthma: causes and diagnosis. *Veterinary Technician the Complete Journal for the Veterinary Hospital Staff* **25**(12): 807-813.

B. Marcucci (2004b) Feline asthma: treatment and prognosis. *Veterinary Technician the Complete Journal for the Veterinary Hospital Staff* **25**(12): 820-826.

S. Marks (2003) Respiratory emergencies. Western Veterinary Conference.

E. Mazzaferro (2003) Respiratory system evaluation and monitoring. American Animal Hospital Association Scientific Program.

M. Tefend (2004) Gussie: a Rottweiler with breathing problems. *Veterinary Technician the Complete Journal for the Veterinary Hospital Staff* **25**(12): 830-834.

Chapter 18
Grasping Gastrointestinal Nursing Care

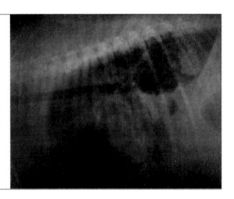

Digestive system

The oral cavity contains the lips, teeth, gingiva, tongue, hard palate, and tonsils. Swallowing begins with the movement of material (bolus) to the back of the mouth and moves toward the pharynx. The pharynx functions in deglutition and serves as a common pathway for food entering the digestive system as well as air entering the lungs. Food then enters the cervical esophagus, which is a muscular tube that carries food via peristalsis to the thoracic esophagus, terminating at the cardia of the stomach (Fig. 18.1).

The stomach functions to store and mix ingesta with secretions, creating a smooth paste. The stomach is a reservoir located in the left side of the abdominal cavity. There are four regions of the stomach: the esophageal; the cardiac (entry); the fundus, which is the true body of the stomach containing gastric glands; and the pylorus (exits). The pylorus is a peristaltic pump that is able to pass the smaller contents to the small intestine. The small intestine is the longest portion of the alimentary canal with two types of motility, segmentation and peristalsis. Segmentation consists of short contractions, while peristalsis is a wave-like contraction. The small intestine consists of the duodenum, the jejunum, and the ilium. The duodenum is the first section of the bowel and controls gastric emptying. The common bile duct, which delivers bile from the gallbladder, and pancreatic duct (delivers enzymes) empty into the duodenum. The jejunum is the longest portion of the small bowel and is freely moveable. The ileum is the shortest portion and it terminates at the ileocecolic junction of the large intestine. The large intestine consists of a cecum, colon, rectum, and anus. The segmental contractions of the colon are called haustral contractions, while mass movement is referred to as peristalic contractions, and finally, filling of the cecum from the colon is termed retrograde contractions. The cecum has no function, while the colon serves to remove water from the stool. The colon has three portions: the ascending, transverse, and descending. The descending colon ends at the rectum, which begins at the pelvic canal. The rectum terminates at the anus, a muscular sphincter (Fig. 18.2).

Clinical Small Animal Care: Promoting Patient Health through Preventative Nursing, First Edition. Kimm Wuestenberg.
© 2012 John Wiley & Sons, Inc. Published 2012 by John Wiley & Sons, Inc.

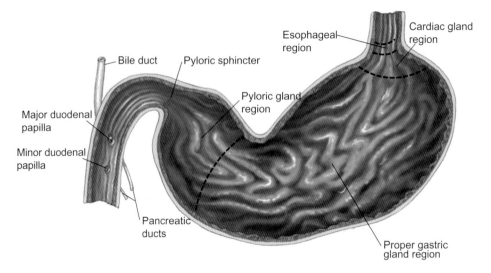

Figure 18.1 Diagram of the stomach. Reproduced with permission from McCracken, T. and Kainer, R. *Color Atlas of Small Animal Anatomy: The Essentials, Revised Edition.* Wiley-Blackwell, 2009.

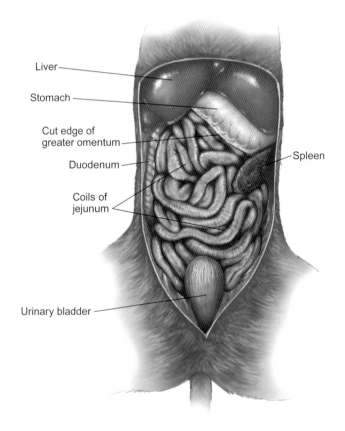

Figure 18.2 Diagram of the abdominal cavity. Reproduced with permission from McCracken, T. and Kainer, R. *Color Atlas of Small Animal Anatomy: The Essentials, Revised Edition.* Wiley-Blackwell, 2009.

There are several accessory glands associated with the digestive system: the salivary glands, liver, gall bladder, and pancreas. The salivary glands produce amylase, an enzyme that breaks down carbohydrates, and lipase, the enzyme that breaks down fat. Saliva serves to lubricate the dry food, clean the coat while grooming, and protect the teeth against decay. Salivation (ptyalism) is controlled by the nervous system.

Liver and gall bladder

The liver is located directly caudal to the diaphragm. In most domestic species, the liver is divided into lobes. The hepatic porta is the portal region that contains the hepatic artery, portal vein, and biliary ducts. The liver cells produce bile acids and bile pigments. Bile acids are necessary for the digestion of fats. Bile pigments give the yellow color. The gallbladder is usually located on the right aspect of the liver, nestled in between lobes. The pancreas is U-shaped with a right and left lobe. The body is the portion closest to the duodenum. The pancreas secretes bicarbonate and enzymes. Bicarbonate neutralizes the acid pH of the ingesta. There are four enzymes secreted: trypsin (protein digestion), amylase (carbohydrate digestion), lipase (fat digestion), and chymotrypsin (protein digestion).

Oral cavity conditions consist of periodontal disease, dysphagia, ulcers, cancers, foreign bodies, and many more. Periodontal disease is common in dogs and cats. A large portion of bacteria in the body originated from the oral cavity. Periodontal disease leads to tooth loss and may be a contributing factor in heart and kidney disease. Fractured teeth with pulp exposure are a site for infection as well as pain since the pulp chamber contains blood supply and nerves (Figs. 18.3–18.5).

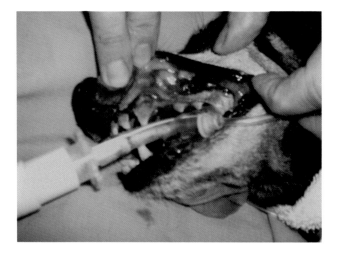

Figure 18.3 Periodontal disease.

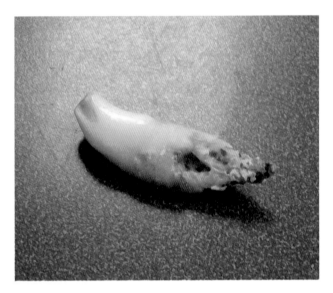

Figure 18.4 Fractured and abscessed canine tooth.

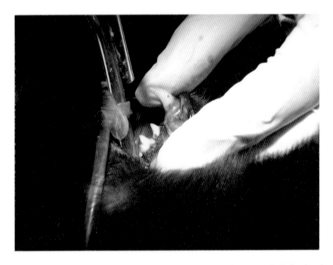

Figure 18.5 Cervical line lesions in lower premolars and enamel defect of canine tooth.

Dysphagia, or difficulty masticating food and swallowing, is frequently associated with neurological conditions. Dysphagia may also lead to an aspiration of food contents into the lungs. Oral ulcers are seen in uremic patients or those who have suffered chemical burn or electrocution. Common cancers of the mouth include melanoma and squamous cell carcinoma. Lastly, foreign bodies such as bones and plant material may cause damage to the gums or teeth and can become lodged in the oral cavity.

Common esophageal conditions include esophagitis, megaesophagus, and strictures. Esophagitis is inflammation of the esophagus and can be due to foreign bodies such as bones, gastric reflux, caustic substances such as chemicals, or *Spirocerca lupi*, an

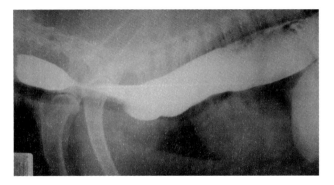

Figure 18.6 Contrast study revealing megaesophagus.

esophageal parasite of the dog. Signs of esophagitis include ptyalism and difficulty swallowing (Fig. 18.6).

Megaesophagus is dilation of the esophagus. The esophagus is a muscle, and when dilated, it loses the ability to adequately move food boluses into the stomach. These patients suffer from regurgitation and are at risk for aspiration pneumonia. Megaesophagus can be congenital as seen in persistent right aortic arch (PRAA), where a stricture is formed around the esophagus by the right aortic arch and the area cranial to the stricture becomes dilated. Megaesophagus can be acquired as seen with myasthenia gravis or a breed disposition as seen in English bulldogs. A stricture is a narrowing of the esophagus, usually occurring as a result of scarring from esophagitis. Large food particles are unable to pass and regurgitation occurs.

Gastric conditions

Vomiting, or emesis, is a contraction of the abdominal wall to empty contents within the stomach. Vomiting is different from regurgitation and reflux in that there is true stomach involvement. Vomiting is controlled by receptors in the stomach and in the brain. Gastritis is a condition in which inflammation of the stomach occurs. Lymphocytic plasmacytic enteritis is a chronic food allergy disorder that is most often seen in cats.

Gastric ulcers may be primary or secondary and cause ulceration of the gastric mucosa. Gastric ulcers can cause hematemesis, but even more severe, perforation of the stomach. Gastric neoplasia can occur, with the most common being gastric lymphoma and gastric adenocarcinoma. These patients often have a history of chronic vomiting and weight loss.

Pyloric outflow problems can occur such as pyloric hypertrophy, a thickening of the pylorus. These patients may have projectile vomiting. It is important to recognize that gastric foreign body obstructions often occur in the pylorus as well (Figs. 18.7-18.10).

Gastric dilatation-volvulus (GDV) is a life-threatening surgical emergency. The stomach rotates, swells, and impedes circulation to the stomach and the caudal vena cava. Symptoms include retching, pacing, panting, abdominal distension, and shock. If left untreated, the symptoms will progress to end-stage shock and death (Tables 18.1 and 18.2, Figs. 18.11 and 18.12).

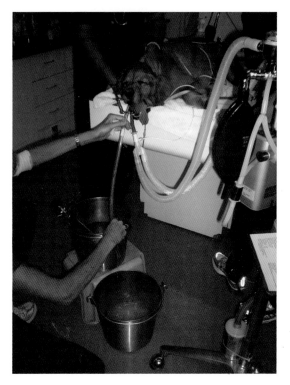

Figure 18.7   Gastric lavage in rodenticide toxicosis.

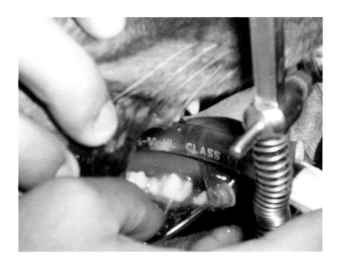

Figure 18.8   Rodenticide ingestion evidenced.

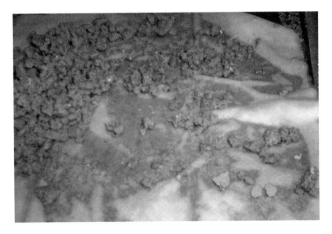

Figure 18.9 Material removed via lavage.

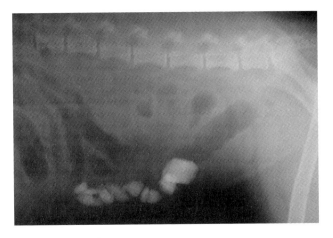

Figure 18.10 Rock foreign body.

Enteric: intestinal disorders

Diarrhea occurs when there is an excess of fluid in the stool. Small bowel diarrhea refers to small intestinal and results in fewer episodes of diarrhea but larger volumes. Large bowel diarrhea, or colonic, is noted by frequent episodes of a small quantity diarrhea. Often mucus and blood is present, along with tenesmus.

Enteritis is an infection or inflammation of the intestines. Many cases are viral such as canine parvovirus and feline panleukopenia, but bacterial infections such as salmonella and campylobacter can also occur. Additionally, protozoal infections such as *Coccidia* and *Giardia* may result in enteritis. Toxicosis and immune-mediated diseases can also cause enteritis (Figs. 18.13–18.15).

Hemorrhagic gastroenteritis or HGE is most common among small breed dogs, particularly Boston terriers and poodles. Symptoms include passing frank bloody diarrhea;

Table 18.1 GDV overview

Stomach expansion	• Rapid accumulation of air • Malposition • With or without volvulus
Stomach rotates 90-270° clockwise	• Distal esophagus/gastroesophageal junction torsion • Air is unable to escape • Fundus of the stomach lies against the ventral abdominal wall • The pylorus moves dorsocranially to the left • Body of stomach moves from left to right side of abdomen • Stomach holds air and fluid • Bacterial formation produces an increase in air
Spleen	• Connected to the stomach by ligaments and vessels • Becomes displaced • May become torsed–secondary splenomegaly
Pressure causes blood flow obstruction	• Abdominal vena cava • Portal vein–hepatic ischemia • Splenic vessels–splenic ischemia
Gastric necrosis	• Leads to grave prognosis
Gastric decompression and shock treatment	• Improves venous return • Improves cardiac output • Improves blood pressure • Shock = tissue hypoxia
Methods of decompression	• Orogastric intubation ("stomach tube") • Gastrocentesis ("trocar")

Table 18.2 Signs and symptoms of GDV

Signs and symptoms of GDV	Common signalment
Panting	Deep-chested dogs
Pacing	Large, giant breeds
Uncomfortable	Can affects smaller breeds
Nonproductive retching	Males appear to be at greater risk
Ptyalism	Increased age = increased risk
Firm, distended abdomen	Highest risk→7-12 years
With or without pulse deficits	Generally over 2 years of age
Shock	Can affect any age

sometimes large clots will be noted. The patients typically have an elevated packed cell volume (PCV) and low protein levels (Table 18.3).

Intussusception is a condition resulting in telescoping of the bowels, with ileum being the common site of the event. This can occur in cases such as canine parvovirus, whipworm infections, and postoperatively with other bowel-related surgeries.

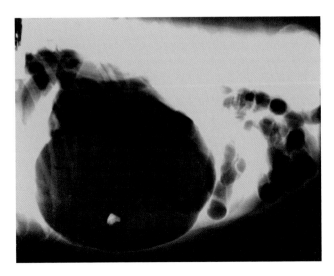

Figure 18.11 GDV with foreign body (rock).

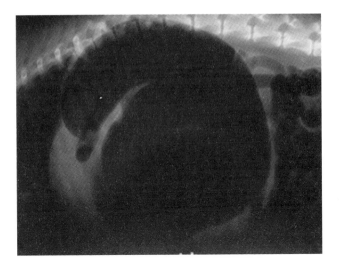

Figure 18.12 Lateral radiograph of GDV.

Malabsorption is a condition in which nutrients are not absorbed through the intestinal mucosa. Diarrhea results from bacterial overgrowth. These animals are usually emaciated and in poor body condition as this is a chronic disease.

Linear foreign bodies occur when an ingested foreign body has the potential to, or does, literally "saw" through the intestines, perforating it. This can be materials such as string or yarn.

Mesenteric torsion occurs when the connective tissue and mesenteric artery that supplies the entire jejunum is twisted (torsed) and obstructs circulation. This is a life-threatening condition requiring surgical correction.

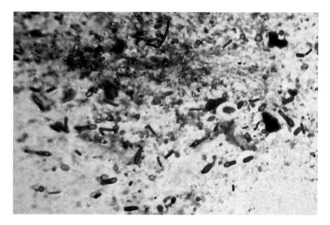

Figure 18.13 Clostridium in fecal cytology.

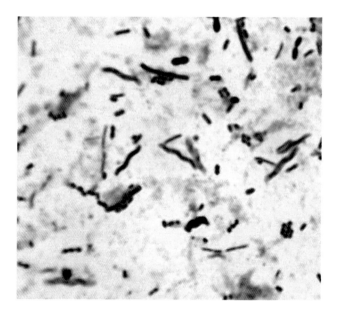

Figure 18.14 Campylobacter in fecal cytology.

Colonic

Colitis, or inflammation or infection of the colon, results in frequent voiding of low volume mucoid to bloody stools. Tenesmus is often present. Causes can include whipworm infection, stress, or diet change. Boxer colitis, however, is an immune-mediated disease similar to Crohn's disease in humans.

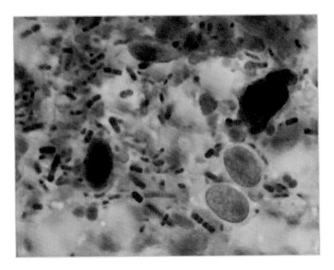

Figure 18.15 Giardia cysts in fecal cytology.

Table 18.3 Types of diarrhea

Osmotic	Additional water pulled into GI tract
Altered mucosal permeability	Inflammatory, infectious, or infiltrative where water (and nutrients) cannot pass through intestinal wall
Abnormal motility	Rapid movement of contents through GI tract
Secretory	Cells of intestinal lining secrete more than they absorb

Pancreatic

Pancreatitis is an inflammation of the pancreas. This is a common disorder in the dog and is becoming more frequently diagnosed in the cat. Symptoms range from gastrointestinal (GI) upset such as anorexia and vomiting to severe hemorrhagic pancreatitis, disseminated intravascular coagulation (DIC), and death. A common cause of pancreatitis is the consumption of a high protein and high fat meal.

Pancreatic insufficiency is less common. Animals suffering from this condition will tend to have soft, greasy, foul-smelling stools. They are often thin animals with poor coats. German Shepherd Dogs (GSDs) are most commonly associated with this disease.

Hepatic

Hepatic conditions include hepatitis, portacaval shunt (PSS), hepatic lipidosis (HL), and hepatobiliary disorders. PSS occurs when the portal vein has diverted blood away from the liver, instead moving it to the vena cava. HL is seen in overweight cats who have

Table 18.4 Clinical signs of liver disease and late-stage liver disease

Clinical signs of liver disease
  Anorexia
  Hiding
  Vomiting
  Diarrhea
  Dehydration
  Weight loss
  Exercise intolerance
  Behavioral changes
  Failure to groom
Late-stage liver disease
  Jaundice
  Effusion

been subjected to a prolonged fasting (or anorexic) period, usually greater than 2–3 days. A sudden diet change in a previously healthy cat can also induce this disease. As the animal fasts, the liver is literally replaced by fat that has been pulled in from adipose tissue. Hepatobiliary disorders involve both the liver and the biliary tract (Table 18.4).

Nursing consideration of patients suffering from GI conditions requires impeccable hygiene, monitoring of excretory losses, and balancing the losses. Excretory losses such as vomit, diarrhea, and urine output should be quantitated and qualitated with a description recorded in the record. Patients suffering from diarrhea should have frequent walks (dog) and fresh litter boxes available for cats. Patients who are eating yet not producing bowel movements should be monitored closely with potential interventions of a diet change or enema administration.

Patients should always be clean of feces, vomit, urine, and so on. If a patient suffers from diarrhea, consider clipping the affected hair to ensure skin is kept clean and monitored for infection. A 10 blade may be beneficial in reducing the risk of clipper-induced skin injury. Protective ointments may be applied once the skin is clean and dry. Areas soiled by vomit such as the muzzle or forelimbs require cleaning. A "bedside" bath can easily be implemented to keep the patient clean.

Other interventions include monitoring electrolyte disturbances, renal function, cardiac arrhythmias (i.e., GDV), DIC (i.e., pancreatitis), or signs of bacterial translocation due to a loss of mucosal integrity of the GI tract, which may result in sepsis, systemic inflammatory response syndrome (SIRS), and multiple organ dysfunction. Ideally, measures would be taken to prevent bacterial translocation, but veterinary personnel should always anticipate this possibility.

Patients with liver disease may only become clinical once the liver reserve capacity has become exhausted. Clinical signs of liver disease may range from vomiting to jaundice, ascites, abnormal bleeding, or even coma (hepatic encephalopathy). When liver disease is present, all major organ systems require clinical monitoring as multiple organ failure is a possible sequela. Fluid balances, respiratory analysis, mentation, and cardio-vascular function are imperative to monitor in anticipation of multiple organ failure. Fluid, electrolyte, and acid-base status should be monitored, as well as signs of bleeding, ascites, and cerebral edema.

Chapter references and further reading

J. Grady (2008) Acute abdominal conditions. International Veterinary Emergency and Critical Care Symposium.

J. Hoskins, et al. (2005) Liver disease in dogs and cats. *Veterinary Technician the Complete Journal for the Veterinary Hospital Staff* **26**(5): 370-377.

J. Kristel (2008) Options for treating a fractured tooth. *Veterinary Technician the Complete Journal for the Veterinary Hospital Staff* **29**(2): 92-99.

C. Lecoindre (2006) Flexible GI endoscopy in cats. *The National Association of Veterinary Technicians in America Journal* **Fall**: 40-45.

E. Mazzaferro (2003) Pre- and post-op management of gastric dilatation-volvulus. American Animal Hospital Association Scientific Program.

K. Michel (2005) Nutrition for patients with acute pancreatitis. *Veterinary Technician the Complete Journal for the Veterinary Hospital Staff* **26**(1): 34-39.

C. Norkus, H. Juda (2005) Gastric dilatation-volvulus. *Veterinary Technician the Complete Journal for the Veterinary Hospital Staff* **26**(4): 269-280.

J. Weese (2008) Beneficial bacteria: a primer on probiotics and GI health. *Veterinary Technician the Complete Journal for the Veterinary Hospital Staff* **29**(6): 332-333.

A. Wortinger (2005) Canine pancreatitis. *The National Association of Veterinary Technicians in America Journal* **Spring**: 37-41.

A. Wortinger (2009) Dealing with diarrhea woes. *Veterinary Technician the Complete Journal for the Veterinary Hospital Staff* **30**(6): 22-28.

Chapter 19
Rendering Renal Care

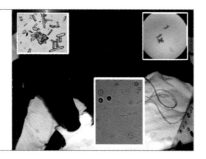

The excretory system

Overview of anatomy and physiology

There are four divisions of the urinary system: the kidneys, ureter, urinary bladder, and urethra (Fig. 19.1). The ultimate function of the kidney is to clean the blood delivered to it of toxic metabolites, help maintain blood pressure by wasting or conserving water and salt, and producing hormones. The kidneys are located in the retroperitoneal space near the spine and are generally easily palpable. In most species, the right kidney is placed cranially and the left kidney is placed caudally. The kidney is divided into three parts: the cortex, medulla, and the pelvis. The nephron is the basic structural and functional unit of the kidney. It is responsible for filtration of the plasma. The vascular portion brings blood to and from the kidney via the glomerulus while the filtration portion filters the plasma, adding or removing water, electrolytes, and toxins from the plasma.

The ureters are structures of tubular smooth muscle that carry the filtrate, or urine, formed by the kidney to the urinary bladder. They enter the bladder near the pelvis in the trigone region. The urinary bladder is a sac-like structure of smooth muscle that has the ability to expand as it becomes filled, then contract to a small size to expel the urine. When empty, the bladder is almost completely in the pelvic cavity.

The urethra is the duct that carries the urine from the bladder to the outside of the body. It is comprised of both smooth and skeletal muscle. The urethra of the male is much longer and narrower than the female, which is why male cats and dogs become obstructed by uroliths more often than females.

Uropoieses is the formation of urine and involves three steps: filtration, reabsorption, and secretion. As blood enters the glomerulus, water, salt, glucose, electrolytes, and amino acids move into the Bowman's capsule and then become what is known as "glomerular filtrate." The glomerular filtration rate (GFR) is the rate at which urine is formed. The GFR is caused by blood pressure. With an increased GFR, there is an

Clinical Small Animal Care: Promoting Patient Health through Preventative Nursing, First Edition. Kimm Wuestenberg.
© 2012 John Wiley & Sons, Inc. Published 2012 by John Wiley & Sons, Inc.

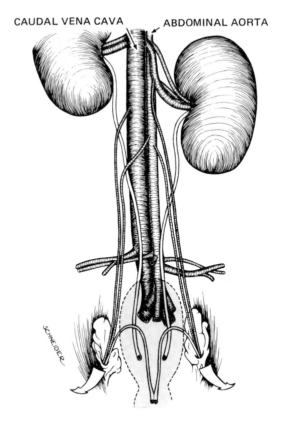

CAUDAL VENA CAVA   ABDOMINAL AORTA

Figure 19.1 Kidneys, ureters, and bladder with surrounding vasculature. Reprinted with permission from Adams, D. *Canine Anatomy: A Systemic Study, Fourth Edition.* Blackwell Publishing, 2004.

increase in pressure, which may be due to overhydration, vasoconstriction, or sodium retention, for example. A decreased GFR is due to decreased pressure, and may be seen in cases of dehydration, vasodilation, or hemorrhage.

Reabsorption occurs in the proximal convoluted tubules and the loop of Henle. Water, bicarbonate, glucose, amino acids, and electrolytes are reabsorbed from the glomerular filtrate into the peritubular capillaries. During secretion, urea is converted to ammonia, while hydrogen conversion depends on the body's needs. Potassium and organic compounds such as medications or toxins are then transported to the distal convoluted tubules (Fig. 19.2).

Hormonal regulation also influences the urinary system. The antidiuretic hormone (ADH), or vasopressin, regulates the reabsorption of water within the kidney (an increase in ADH will cause an increase in water reabsorption in the kidney). Aldosterone is a hormone that stimulates sodium reabsorption in the kidney. An increase in sodium leads to water retention and increased water retention leads to increased blood pressure. It also acts as a vasoconstrictor, which will increase blood pressure. The regulation of sodium and blood pressure is thus dependent on hormone regulation. Micturition, or voiding of the bladder, is under the influence of neurological controls. There are two

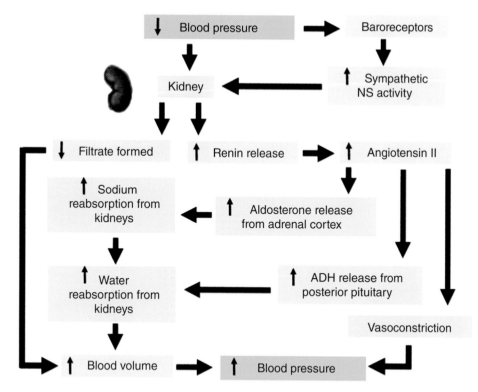

Figure 19.2 Renin-angiotensis system diagram. NS, nervous system. Reprinted with permission from Akers, M. and Denbow, M. e. Wiley-Blackwell, 2008.

valves located at the top of the urethra: the internal smooth muscle sphincter, which is involuntary, and the external sphincter, which is voluntary.

Renal injury occurs in three ways: prerenal, which occurs before filtration, renal, and postrenal, involving the urinary tract. Prerenal includes poor renal blood flow conditions such as dehydration, shock, or low blood volume. Renal conditions involve the kidneys in either acute or chronic failure. Acute renal failure (ARF) symptoms include oliguria or anuria, enlarged kidneys, and a rapid decline in renal function. ARF can be caused by toxins, heatstroke, diabetes mellitus (DM), and other metabolic diseases. Chronic renal failure (CRF) is seen in elderly, dehydrated animals. They often have a history of weight loss, excessive water drinking, and urination. Animals with CRF will produce large volumes of urine and have small kidneys, as opposed to ARF. The cause of CRF can be unknown, due to a kidney infection or from chronic toxicity to the kidney. Nephritis is a degenerative condition of the nephrons, which is a common cause of CRF. Low protein diets are recommended for patients with renal injury, as this reduces the work-load of the kidneys. Anemia may also be seen as the kidneys produce the hormone erythropoietin.

Postrenal injury occurs as a result of lower urinary tract perforation or obstruction. Urinary tract obstruction, or UTO, occurs when small crystals form in the urine, creating calculi or uroliths that prevent the outflow of urine from the bladder. The obstruction

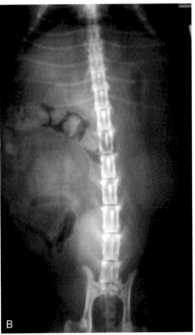

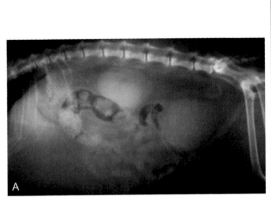

Figures 19.3 Lateral (A) and ventrodorsal (B) radiograph views of enlarged kidney and bladder in a male cat with UTO.

can occur in the bladder or urethra, although kidney stones may result in an obstructed ureter. When the urethra is obstructed, the bladder continues to enlarge due to urine production, but the urine cannot be expelled. The bladder can rupture and the patient can succumb to severe metabolic disturbances such as hyperkalemia. Symptoms may include a tense, painful abdomen, straining, or vocalizing upon urination, hematuria, and frequent episodes of scant urine. Males are most commonly affected by urinary obstructions due to the narrow urethra when compared to the female urethra. Immediate treatment establishing a patent urine outflow is imperative to prevent toxic buildup in the body and bladder rupture (Figs. 19.3-19.5).

Other urinary conditions include glomerular nephritis, which is an immune-mediated destruction of the glomerulus; pyelonephritis, which is a bacterial or yeast infection in the kidney; and polycystic renal disease, a heritable congenital disease where large, fluid-filled cysts occupy the kidney. Hydronephrosis is a condition in which the renal pelvis is stretched and distended with fluid (urine) and eventually the tissue becomes fibrosed.

Urogenital conditions

Dystocia is one of the most common emergencies of the reproductive system (Figs. 19.6 and 19.7). Dystocia is having a difficult (or impossible) delivery. Factors include fetal size and position, uterine inertia, exhaustion, and premature placental separation in

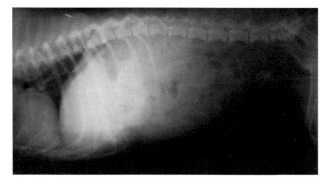

Figure 19.4 Lateral radiograph of nephrolith, ureterlith, and uroliths.

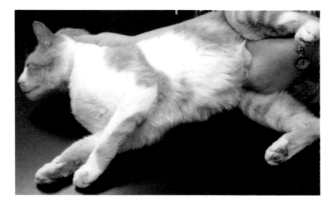

Figure 19.5 Bladder palpation technique in a cat.

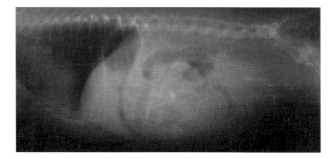

Figure 19.6 Lateral radiograph.

addition to metabolic disturbances. History will usually include prolonged laboring without the production of offspring, straining, panting, anxiety, and possibly inappetance or vomiting.

A pyometra is a large, purulent uterus. It is very common in the dog, especially the older female. There are two classifications for pyometra, open and closed. In an open pyometra, the cervix is open and able to drain, creating a foul-smelling bloody

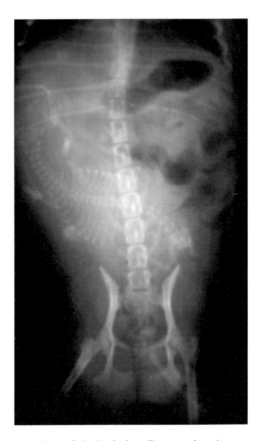

Figure 19.7   Venrodorsal view of dystocia in a Pomeranian dog.

discharge, usually postestrous cycle. In a closed pyometra, the cervix is closed, creating a very large, toxic uterus. Symptoms for both classifications include lethargy, vomiting, leukocytosis (seen in early-to-middle-stage pyometra), or leukopenia (seen in late stage, usually due to sepsis); an open pyometra will have a discharge. Radiographs will show an enlarged uterus (Fig. 19.8).

Uterine prolapse occurs when the uterine is expelled out of the body through the vagina. It can often accompany dystocia. Clinical signs include the presence of the uterus, usually with a history of recent parturition.

Nursing interventions

Patients with renal compromise require astute monitoring of fluid balances. Fluid balances primarily include quantitating fluid therapy delivery and urine output. If a chest tube or peritoneal dialysis tube is in place, the fluid obtained from the chest tube should be included, as well as the fluid administered and aspirated from peritoneal dialysis. Any fluid losses from vomiting or diarrhea should also be calculated. Patients should also be weighed, at minimum every 12 hours. In severe cases, monitoring weight may

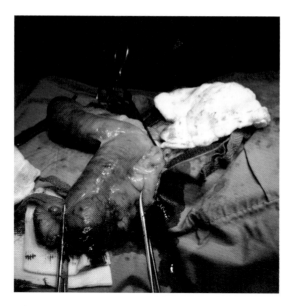

Figure 19.8 Pyometra.

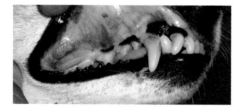

Figure 19.9 Uremic ulcers in an azotemic dog.

be necessary every 2–4 hours. When the kidneys are impaired, the patient may retain excess fluid, resulting in edema of the limbs and fluid accumulation in body cavities. This occurrence is often referred to as "third spacing." It may be beneficial to place an indwelling urinary catheter to aid in accurate balancing. Patients at bare minimum should produce 1–2 mL of urine per pound per hour. Patients with urine output below this rate should be assessed for additional therapy. Diuretics or medications to dilate the renal arteries, promoting blood flow to the kidney, may be warranted. Body weight assessment and fluid balance intervals may need to be increased. The patient with renal failure should also be assessed for mental status as multiple organ dysfunction can quickly ensue as the kidneys further deteriorate. The patient should also be assessed for oral ulceration (uremic ulcers) and frequent oral rinses should be scheduled to aid in oral health. A typical renal diet is low in protein to reduce the workload of the kidneys (Figs. 19.9–19.11).

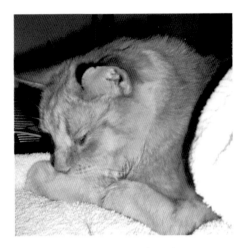

Figure 19.10 Neck ventroflexion in a hypokalemic cat.

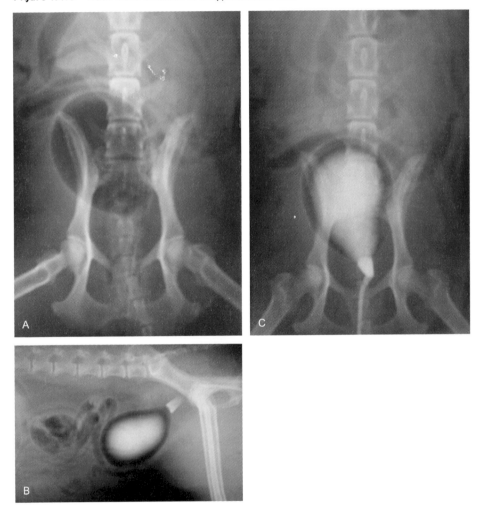

Figure 19.11 Bladder study. A. Ventrodorsal view of a pneumocystogram (negative contrast study). B. Lateral view of a double-contrast cystogram. C. Ventrodorsal view of double-contrast cystogram. These studies are useful in identification of masses, calculi, or rupture.

Chapter references and further reading

C. Adams (2008) Updates in management of chronic kidney disease. *The National Association of Veterinary Technicians in America Journal* **Summer**: 43-48.

G. Grauer (2003a) Preventing acute renal failure. American Animal Hospital Association Scientific Program.

G. Grauer (2003b) Management of complications of feline chronic renal failure. American Animal Hospital Association Scientific Program.

M. Kerl (2008) Renal failure in cats: new concepts. International Veterinary Emergency and Critical Care Symposium.

I. Lane (2003a) Renal failure in cats I and II. Western Veterinary Conference.

I. Lane (2003b) Upper tract uroliths in cats. Western Veterinary Conference.

J. Lulich (2003) Managing reversible renal failure I and II. Western Veterinary Conference.

P. Matthews (2005) A dog with transitional cell carcinoma. *Veterinary Technician the Complete Journal for the Veterinary Hospital Staff* **26**(5): 220-221.

T. Rieser (2003a) Canine and feline urethral obstructions. Western Veterinary Conference.

T. Rieser (2003b) Acute renal failure. Western Veterinary Conference.

T. Rieser (2008) Renal emergencies: diagnosis and treatment. International Veterinary Emergency and Critical Care Symposium.

S. Ross (2003) Renal and ureteral urolithiasis. American Animal Hospital Association Scientific Program.

K. Stafford (2004) Enhanced radiographic studies. *Veterinary Technician the Complete Journal for the Veterinary Hospital Staff* **25**(6): 384-393.

Chapter 20
Endocrine Nursing Encounters

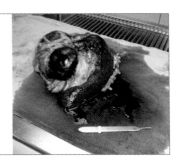

The endocrine system

Hormones are control chemicals that are produced, stored, and released by specialized glands in the body and have a specific effect on certain target tissues. The endocrine system functions in communication, coordination, and control, and often works together with the nervous system. There are 13 endocrine glands in the mammal.

The pituitary, or "master gland," is located in the base of the brain and has three divisions: the anterior, intermediate, and posterior lobes. The anterior lobe produces growth hormone (GH), prolactin (PRL), thyroid-stimulating hormone (TSH), adrenocorticotropic hormone (ACTH), follicle-stimulating hormone (FSH), and luteinizing hormone (LH). The intermediate lobe produces melanocyte-stimulating hormone (MSH) and the posterior lobe produces oxytocin and antidiuretic hormone (ADH), in addition to acting as a storage area for the hormones produced by the hypothalamus.

The thyroid glands are two glands located in the neck region, just caudal to the larynx. They produce triiodothyronine (T_3), thyroxin (T_4), and calcitonin, and store iodine. Triiodothyronine targets most tissues and is necessary for the proper function of the nervous and muscular systems. Triiodothyronine also influences protein synthesis and growth. Both triiodothyronine and thyroxin stimulate metabolism. Calcitonin works to prevent excess calcium by removing the excess calcium out of the serum, preventing gastrointestinal absorption of calcium and excreting excess calcium via renal tubules. The thyroid gland targets bone as a storage area for calcium.

The parathyroid is located near the thyroid gland and produces the hormone parathormone. Parathormone regulates calcium and phosphorus levels and targets the bone, kidney, and intestines. It releases calcium from the bones, promotes the absorption of calcium from the gastrointestinal system, and promotes the absorption of calcium while preventing phosphorus absorption in the renal tubules. All of these functions together increase serum calcium levels, having the exact opposite effect of

Clinical Small Animal Care: Promoting Patient Health through Preventative Nursing, First Edition.
Kimm Wuestenberg.
© 2012 John Wiley & Sons, Inc. Published 2012 by John Wiley & Sons, Inc.

calcitonin. The amount of parathormone secreted is regulated by the level of calcium in extracellular fluid.

The endocrine glands of the digestive system include the stomach, the duodenum, and the pancreas. The hormone produced in the stomach is gastrin. Gastrin is stimulated by proteins entering the stomach and then releases hydrochloric acid and pepsinogen. Gastrin also stimulates the pancreas to increase insulin production and the liver to increase bile production. The duodenum produces three hormones: secretin, cholecystokinin, and inerogastrone. Secretin stimulates pancreatic enzymes to neutralize the stomach acidity of chyme, while inerogastrone, which is stimulated by fat, inhibits gastric secretions and mobility, keeping chyme in the stomach longer so the fat has the opportunity to be broken down. The hormone cholecystokinin stimulates the gallbladder to release bile into the duodenum. The pancreas contains the islets of Langerhans, which are a small cluster of cells that release the hormones glucagon and insulin.

Glucogon stimulates the formation of glucose by converting liver glycogen to glucose. It prevents the insulin from lowering the blood sugar too low, thus preventing hypoglycemia. Insulin converts glucose to glycogen, lowering the blood glucose levels.

The adrenal glands are a pair of glands located just cranial to each kidney. There are two regions: the interior portion called the adrenal medulla, and the exterior portion called the adrenal cortex. The adrenal medulla is a true endocrine gland, but is also considered part of the nervous system. Epinephrine and norepinephrine are the hormones produced in the adrenal medulla. Epinephrine stimulates adrenaline, or a sympathetic response. Norepinephrine causes vasoconstriction, increasing blood pressure. Both of these hormones target the heart, vessels, and most other tissues. The adrenal cortex contains glucocorticoids (cortisone and cortisol), which increase blood glucose and metabolize fat and protein. Mineralocorticoids are also found in the adrenal cortex. Aldosterone targets the kidney and stimulates water and sodium retention. Sex hormones responsible for secondary sex characteristics are also located here. The kidneys also produce two hormones, renin and erythropoietin. Renin causes an increased blood pressure by the action of the adrenal cortex, and erythropoietin is the hormone that stimulates red blood cell production.

Additional endocrine glands include the ovaries, which produce estrogen and progesterone; the testes, which produce testosterone; the thymus, which stimulates immunity in the young; the pineal gland, which produces melatonin and regulates gonadotropins; and lastly, the placenta, which produces hormones that maintain pregnancy in some species (Fig. 20.1).

Endocrine diseases are classified as "hyper" or "hypo," either too much production of a hormone or not enough production. Hormones need to bind to a receptor to function, therefore occasionally there is adequate hormone but the receptor is not functioning (Fig. 20.2).

Adrenal gland disease is primarily a canine disease. Hyperadrenocorticism or hyperadrenocortisolism (Cushing's disease) occurs when excess cortisol is produced by the adrenal gland. These dogs typically have a barrel body with thin legs, a pot-bellied appearance with hair loss, and rough skin. There are changes in fat storage and poor wound healing occurs. They are generally polydipsic and polyuric. Cushing's can be pituitary dependent, caused by an adrenal tumor or iatrogenic.

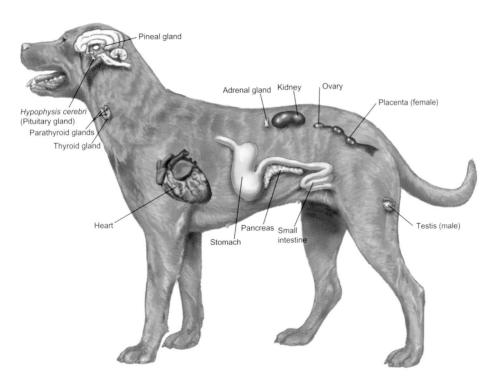

Figure 20.1 Location of major endocrine organs. Reprinted with permission from McCracken, T. and Kainer, R. *Color Atlas of Small Animal Anatomy: The Essentials, Revised Edition.* Wiley-Blackwell, 2009

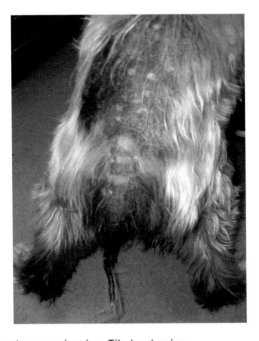

Figure 20.2 Hyperadrenocorcism in a Tibetan terrier.

Hypoadrenocorticism or hypoadrenocortisolism (Addison's disease) can cause low blood pressure due to hyperkalemia, anorexia, and muscle weakness. Symptoms reported by owners are usually episodes of intermittent anorexia, vomiting, diarrhea, weight loss, and a change in hair coat. An Addisonian crisis is a severe, life-threatening hyperkalemia, leading to bradycardia and shock.

Common thyroid gland disorders include hypothyroidism and hyperthyroidism. Hypothyroidism primarily affects dogs and results in clinical signs such as obesity, lethargy, skin, and hair coat abnormalities such as rough, brittle hair and thick, heavy skin. Hyperthyroidism primarily affects cats and is relatively rare in dogs but can occur with malignant thyroid cancer in dogs. Hyperthyroidism signs include weight loss, irritability, and the pet may be hyperactive.

Diabetes mellitus (DM) affects both dogs and cats, among other species. A lack of insulin production by the pancreas causes blood glucose levels to elevate. Signs include weight loss, polydipsia, polyuria, and polyphagia. Vomiting and lethargy may also accompany DM. Diabetic ketoacidosis (DKA or diabetic crisis) is a severe metabolic condition that occurs in unregulated patients with diabetes who remain hyperglycemic. The patients may suffer from anorexia, vomiting, diarrhea, severe dehydration, and typically have ketonuria and extremely high blood glucose levels. These patients are critical, often presenting comatose or near comatose and require medical management to correct the metabolic abnormalities.

Diabetes insipidus is caused by a lack of ADH, and excessive loss of fluid coupled with retention of sodium. Water is not being reabsorbed, polydipsia is present, and large amounts of water are excreted in the urine, causing a decreased urine specific gravity.

Since endocrine disorders can be due to many aspects of the body, such as adrenal, pancreatic, and thyroid disorders, nursing care can be widespread, from monitoring for signs of hypercalcemia to hypoglycemia. General body functions such as organ systems and laboratory values should be assessed, as well as implementing applied patient care such as fluid balancing, hygiene, and intense monitoring in anticipation of disease progression (Tables 20.1 and 20.2).

Table 20.1 Endocrine disorders and symptoms

Condition	Commonly associated clinical symptoms
Adrenal	
Hypoadrenocorticism (Addison's disease)	Weight loss, anorexia, weakness, lethargy, collapse, muscle fasciculations, intermittent vomiting, diarrhea, melena or hematochezia, polyuria, polydipsia.
	Addisonian crisis: hypovolemic shock, bradycardia
Hyperadrenocorticism (Cushing's disease)	Polyuria, polydipsia, polyphagia, bilateral symmetrical alopecia, thin skin, hyperpigmentation of skin, pendulous abdominal distension
Pheochromocytoma	Tachycardia, tachypnea, severe hypertension (retinal detachment, cardiac arrhythmias, hyperemic skin, etc.), shock

Table 20.1 (*Continued*)

Condition	Commonly associated clinical symptoms
Pancreatic	
DM	Polydipsia, polyuria, polyphagia, weight loss, cataract formation, lethargy, muscle atrophy
DKA	Anorexia, vomiting, acetone odor of breath, depressed, obtunded or comatose, icterus
Insulinoma	Weakness, ataxia, seizures, muscle fasciculations, polyphagia
Thyroid	
Myxedema coma	Bradycardia, hypothermia, thickened skin, nonpitting edema, decreased level of consciousness (LOC), hypoventilation
Thyroid storm	Severe hyperthermia, cardiac arrhythmias, vomiting, stupor, coma
Parathyroid	
Hypoparathyroidism	Aggression, facial rubbing, panting, nervousness, muscle fasciculations, tetany, generalized, seizures, weakness, lethargy and anorexia
Hyperparathyroidism	Polyuria, polydipsia, dysuria, pollakiuria, hematuria, anorexia, vomiting, constipation

Table 20.2 Splenic conditions

Splenic torsion	Associated with gastric dilatation-volvulus (GDV)
Splenomegaly	Inflammatory, hyperplastic, congestive, infiltrative
Trauma	Blunt or penetrating
Splenic masses	Neoplastic or benign

Chapter references and further reading

E. Behrend (2003) Diabetes insipidus and other causes of polyuria/polydipsia. Western Veterinary Conference.

A. Breton (2005) The spleen anatomy and common complications. *Veterinary Technician the Complete Journal for the Veterinary Hospital Staff* **26**(8): 554-564.

D. Elliot (2005) Feline diabetes mellitus. *The National Association of Veterinary Technicians in America Journal* **Fall**: 36-41.

S. Krick (2002) Understanding hypothyroidism. *Veterinary Technician the Complete Journal for the Veterinary Hospital Staff* **23**(10): 634-636.

S. Krick (2003a) Understanding Cushing's disease in dogs. *Veterinary Technician the Complete Journal for the Veterinary Hospital Staff* **24**(1): 40-42.

S. Krick (2003b) Understanding diabetes mellitus. *Veterinary Technician the Complete Journal for the Veterinary Hospital Staff* **24**(2): 123-127.

T. Rieser (2003) Initial treatment of diabetic ketoacidosis. Western Veterinary Conference.

M. Schaer (2003) Endocrine emergencies. Western Veterinary Conference.

B. Tabor (2008) Understanding and treating diabetic ketoacidosis. *Veterinary Technician the Complete Journal for the Veterinary Hospital Staff* **29**(4): 227-233.

L. Williams, R. Bagely (1998) Diagnosing and managing canine hyperadrenocorticism. *Veterinary Technician the Complete Journal for the Veterinary Hospital Staff* **19**(1): 47-56.

Chapter 21
Nursing Care of the Neurological Patient

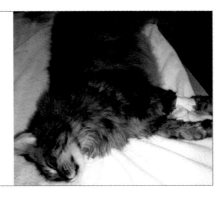

Nervous system

The nervous system is a communication network with three basic functions of sensing, integrating, and motor. The sensory portion of the nervous system detects change in the body while the integrating aspect analyzes and responds to information received. The motor response commands muscles to move or for glands to respond by producing secretions.

There are two types of cells in the nervous system: glial cells (nonneuronal), which support and protect the nervous system, and neurons, which transmit information and impulses. Afferent nerves are those that conduct impulses toward the central nervous system (CNS) and efferent nerves conduct impulses away from the CNS (Figs. 21.1 and 21.2).

The CNS is made up of the brain and spinal cord. The meninges cover the brain and spinal cord and are made up of three layers: the pia mater (inner layer), the arachnoid (middle layer), and the dura mater (outer layer). Cerebral spinal fluid (CSF) circulates between the layers of the meninges and cushions the brain as well as regulating the extracellular brain fluid The brain has four sections: the cerebrum, the cerebellum, the diencephalons, and the brain stem. The cerebrum is the largest part of the brain and is considered the highest center, the portion of conscious thought, and perception of sensations. The cerebellum is the portion of the brain that controls motor function. The diencephalon is made up of the thalamus, hypothalamus, and pituitary. While the thalamus functions in sensory impulses and consciousness, the hypothalamus is a communication center for both the nervous system and the endocrine system. The pituitary is often referred to as "the master gland," as it is involved with hormones, temperature regulation, hunger and thirst, and anger regulation. The brain stem connects the brain to the spinal cord and is made up of the medulla oblongata, the pons, and the midbrain. Many of the cranial nerves originate in the brain stem and autonomic control of the cardiovascular and pulmonary system is also located here (Fig. 21.3).

Clinical Small Animal Care: Promoting Patient Health through Preventative Nursing, First Edition.
Kimm Wuestenberg.
© 2012 John Wiley & Sons, Inc. Published 2012 by John Wiley & Sons, Inc.

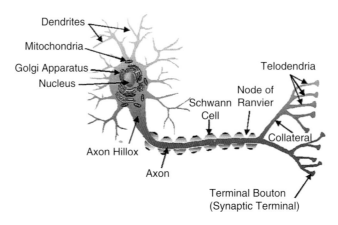

Figure 21.1 Diagram of a typical neuron. Reprinted with permission from Akers, M. and Denbow, M. *Anatomy and Physiology of Domestic Animals*. Wiley-Blackwell, 2008.

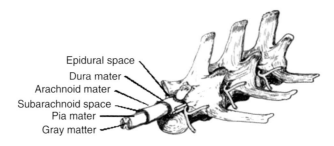

Figure 21.2 Meningeal layers. Reprinted with permission from Akers, M. and Denbow, M. *Anatomy and Physiology of Domestic Animals*. Wiley-Blackwell, 2008.

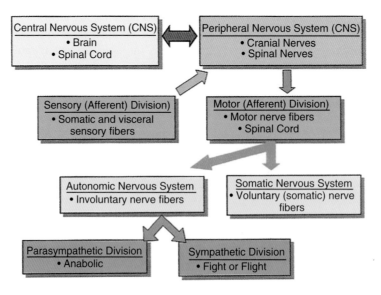

Figure 21.3 CNS and PNS organization. Reprinted with permission from Akers, M. and Denbow, M. *Anatomy and Physiology of Domestic Animals*. Wiley-Blackwell, 2008.

Table 21.1 Cranial nerves

Cranial nerve	Name	Function
I	Olfactory	Sensory neurons for smell
II	Optic	Sensory neurons for sight
III	Oculomotor	Motor nerve for most of the muscles of the eye
IV	Trochlear	Motor nerve that supplies the dorsal oblique muscle of the eye
V	Trigeminal	Mixed nerves; sensory: eye and face; motor: mastication
VI	Abducens	Motor nerve that supplies the retractor and lateral rectus muscles of the eye
VII	Facial	Mixed nerves; sensory: cranial 2/3 for taste; motor: facial expressions and muscles of the ear
VIII	Acoustic	Sensory nerves for hearing and equilibrium (vestibular dz)
IX	Glossopharyngeal	Mixed nerves; sensory: pharynx and caudal 1/3 of the tongue for taste; motor: muscles of the pharynx (swallowing)
X	Vagus	Mixed nerves; sensory: pharynx and larynx; motor: heart, lungs and muscles of the larynx. The vagus nerve is the longest cranial nerve; it runs throughout the thorax and the abdomen.
XI	Spinal accessory	Motor nerve that supplies the muscles of the shoulder and neck
XII	Hypoglossal	Motor nerve that controls the muscles of the tongue

The peripheral nervous system (PNS) is made up of sensory neurons. Stimulus receptors inform the CNS of stimuli and then motor neurons travel from the CNS to the muscles and glands, which ultimately take action or respond to the stimuli. The PNS is made up 12 pairs of cranial nerves, which originate in the brain, and 31 spinal nerves, which originate in the spinal cord. Unlike the cranial nerves, all of the spinal nerves are mixed, meaning they contain both sensory and motor neurons (Table 21.1, Fig. 21.4).

The autonomic nervous system (ANS) is made up of motor and sensory nerves and has automatic functions. The ANS divides into two separate portions, the sympathetic and parasympathetic nervous systems. The sympathetic nervous system, also referred to as adrenergic, controls the "fight-or-flight" response. In extreme stress, the nerve endings of the sympathetic nervous system release epinephrine, which results in physiological changes of an increased heart rate, blood pressure and respiration, bronchodilation and mydriasis, and finally, slowing of gastrointestinal (GI) activity. The parasympathetic nervous system is one of cholinergic affects and controls the normal

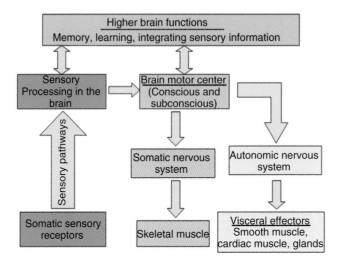

Figure 21.4 Integration of somatic and atonomic nervous systems. Reprinted with permission from Akers, M. and Denbow, M. *Anatomy and Physiology of Domestic Animals*. Wiley-Blackwell, 2008.

homeostatic mechanisms of the body. Parasympathetic nerve fibers release acetylcholine, which causes an opposite effect than that of the sympathetic nervous system. A parasympathetic response results in decreased heart rate, respirations, GI activity, and anal sphincter tone while increasing respiratory and salivary secretions, as well as miosis.

The somatic nervous system is one of conscious, voluntary functions. It is made up of motor and sensory nerves. Communication occurs through the actions of the sodium-potassium pump. Sodium is constantly being moved out of the cell, while potassium is brought back in to the cell. This process is always active, even during the resting phase of transmission. The cell has a negative charge on the inside (potassium) and a positive charge on the outside (sodium), causing an electrical charge across the cell membrane. Depolarization is the stimulation of the nerve and occurs when the sodium channels open, allowing the ions to flow into the cell. This creates a positive electrical charge. During repolarization, the sodium channels close while potassium channels open. Potassium is brought back into the cell while sodium is forced out, creating a negatively charged cell. Not every depolarization stimulus results in a complete cycle. The stimulus must be strong enough to cause complete depolarization. If the stimulus is not strong enough (threshold not met), the active pump would just move the small number of sodium ions back out of the cell. If more channels open and more sodium ions enter the cell, then depolarization would occur and threshold will be met. There is an "all-or-nothing" principle in that the neuron either depolarizes to complete maximum, or it does not depolarize at all. The threshold has to be met in order to depolarize. The refractory phase occurs when the cells cannot respond to new stimuli because they are in the process of repolarizing. Saltatory conduction is a rapid "leaping" conduction that occurs because the myelin sheath has a protective barrier that does not allow sodium within. In this type of nervous tissue conduction, the depolarization wave will occur in

Table 21.2 Synapse function

Presynaptic neuron	Releases a chemical to stimulate the next nerve cell
Neurotransmitter	Chemical transmitted between nerve cells
Excitatory	Causes an influx of sodium, causing a reach in threshold (depolarization)
Inhibitory	Keeps the cell from reaching threshold (depolarization) by bringing chloride into the cell
Postsynaptic neuron	Receives the neurotransmitter
Synaptic end	Found on the axon of the presynaptic neuron; it contains mitochondria for the process
Receptors	Specific areas on the postsynaptic membrane that will allow certain transmitters to bind

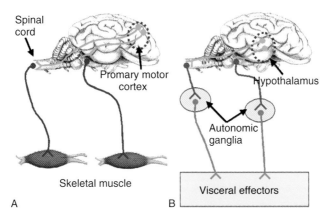

Figure 21.5 Organization of (A) somatic and (B) autonomic nervous systems. Reprinted with permission from Akers, M. and Denbow, M. *Anatomy and Physiology of Domestic Animals*. Wiley-Blackwell, 2008.

the nodes of Ranvier, skipping from one node of Ranvier to the next, and continuing on with the wave becoming accelerated, making transmission very rapid (Table 21.2, Fig. 21.5).

Diseases of the nervous system can be central (CNS), peripheral (PNS), or both. A very common CNS disorder is a seizure. Seizures are transient disturbances of brain function. They have a sudden onset of convulsions and then the seizure ceases spontaneously. There are several classifications and causes of seizure activity (Table 21.3).

Neoplastic brain tumors can occur in many locations of the brain. They may be benign or malignant. Meningioma is a benign growth of the meninges. The growth often places pressure on the brain and spinal cord and causes serious signs such as paralysis or blindness. Encephalitis occurs when there is infection of the brain; it can be viral, fungal, or bacterial in nature. Symptoms of encephalitis include nervous irritation, muscle

Table 21.3 Seizures

Type	Description
Grand mal	Generalized seizure; cerebral in origin. There are no localizing signs; the animal loses consciousness, generalized muscle activity, ptyalism, chewing, opisthotonos, paddling, and urination and defecation.
Petit mal	A mild and brief generalized seizure. Less violent than grand mal
Focal	Partial seizure; a seizure restricted to a focal area of the brain and signs will correspond to the affected area. Localized region: tremors in one limb, "bubble gum" chewing, fly biting, behavioral changes, and episodes of blindness.
Tonic-clonic	Alternating from rigidity (tonic) to jerking movements (clonic)
Cluster seizures	Frequent episodes of seizure activity
Status epilepticus	Sustained seizure; these are medical emergencies as body temperatures can elevate to fatal
Causes	
Metabolic causes	Hypoglycemia (insulinoma)
	Hypocalcemia (eclampsia)
	Hypomagnesemia
	Toxins (rodenticides, insecticides, mycotoxins, scorpion envenomation)
	Hypoxia (asphyxiation)
Physical causes	Tumors (brain tumor, cyst on the brain)
	Ischemia (CVA, aneurysm)
Idiopathic epilepsy	A seizure disorder of unknown origin. It is a heritable disorder in many breeds. Usually epileptics will have their first seizure before the age of 4.

tremors, convulsions, weakness, paralysis, and coma or death. Canine distemper virus (CDV), "old dog encephalitis" (residual CDV encephalitis), granulomatous meningoen-cephalitis/myelitis (GME), and Pug Dog encephalitis (PDE), which is seen in young Pugs, are all encephalitides. Metabolic disorders such as hypoglycemia can also result in seizure activity. Hepatic encephalitis occurs in states of severe liver disease where ammonia levels in the blood and other toxins travel to the brain. Hepatic encephalitis can occur in conditions such as portosystemic shunt (PSS), hepatitis, and hepatic lipidosis. Cerebellar disorders are typically accompanied by symptoms such as intention tremors, hypermetric gait, ataxia, nystagmus, and menace deficits. In pure cerebellar disease, mentation is normal. The causes can be congenital, acute, infectious, degenerative, cystic, or neoplastic in nature. Cerebellar hypoplasia is a congenital disorder seen in kittens born to a cat infected with panleukopenia. Acute injuries such as cerebral vascular accident (CVA) or trauma and infectious agents like feline infectious peritonitis (FIP) or toxoplasmosis can also lead to cerebellar hypoplasia.

Spinal cord diseases can occur due to trauma, such as fracture, Schiff-Sherrington phenomenon, or intervertebral disk disease (IVDD). Schiff-Sherrington phenomenon or syndrome results from a lesion between C3 and T2, usually due to trauma. The result is front-end extensor rigidity while the hind end of the animal is paretic. These animals are typically in pain and treatment will be based on the nature of the lesion. IVDD occurs when the cartilaginous disk(s) between the vertebras become displaced. This condition is common among chondrodystrophic breeds. IVDD can be caused by degeneration, extrusion, protrusion, or herniation of disk material. Fibrocartilagenous embolism (FCE) occurs when intervertebral disk material has been extruded and forced into the meninges or intramedullary blood vessels. It causes an acute paresis or paralysis and treatment generally involves medical management. Meningitis is another spinal cord disease. Inflammation of the meninges can be caused by viral infections, bacterial infections, fungi, chemical, or metastatic malignant cells. Signs of meningitis include fever, hyperesthesia, muscle rigidity, pain, and recumbency. Supportive care is implemented and can be long term while the underlying cause is treated. Cervical spondylomyelopathy, also known as "Wobbler syndrome," occurs with anatomical abnormalities which result in spinal cord compression. This condition can be hereditary and is seen more frequently in Great Danes, Dobermans, and Rottweilers. Symptoms of Wobbler syndrome include cervical neck pain, uncoordinated gait, carrying the head low/reluctant to extend neck, ataxia of the hind limbs, loss of muscle tone, and tetraparesis.

Conditions of the peripheral nerves can be traumatic or acquired. Traumatic injuries commonly seen include brachial plexus avulsion and single nerve injuries. Brachial plexus avulsion is most often seen following a motor vehicle accident. The animal is bumped in the shoulder by the car (brachial plexus) and subsequent radial nerve damage occurs. The limb will lack sensation, it is often dragged when walking, and some animals will chew at the limb. The nerve damage may be temporary or permanent. Many of these cases require amputation. Sciatic nerve injury can be caused by improper intramuscular (IM) injections. The animal may limp or, in severe case, be unable to extend the knee, flex the hock, or bear weight. Radial nerve injuries can accompany a humeral fracture, but may also be caused by improper tourniquet technique. Acquired neuropathies include polyradiculoneuritis, Horner's syndrome, vestibular disease, and myasthenia gravis. Polyradiculoneuritis, formerly called "Coonhound paralysis," was thought to be associated with raccoon saliva but newer cases have proved otherwise. Polyradiculoneuritis is a progressive weakness of the limbs that may progress to quadriplegia. In rare, severe cases, respiratory paralysis occurs and death ensues. Patients can require several months of supportive care for full recovery. Tick bite paralysis is similar to polyradiculoneuritis but is caused by a tick. Upon removing the tick, recovery will usually occur within 24-48 hours. However, supportive care may be needed for an additional 3-4 weeks. Horner's syndrome is a condition that can be peripheral or central in nature. Symptoms include enophthalmus, ptosis, and miosis (Fig. 21.6). Vestibular disease presents with head tilt, circling-falling-paddling, nystagmus, and is usually accompanied by anxiety and nausea.

Vestibular disease can be caused by brain lesions, inner ear infections, or may be idiopathic ("old dog vestibular") (Fig. 21.7).

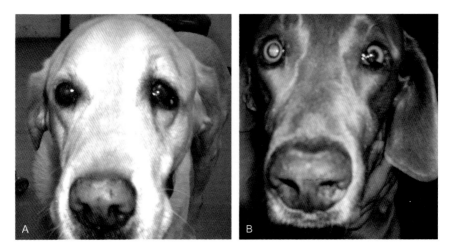

Figures 21.6 Horner's syndrome in (A) a Labrador retriever and (B) a Weimaraner.

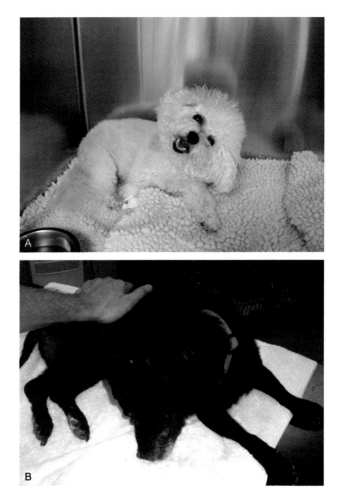

Figures 21.7 Vestibular disease in (A) a Bichon Frise and (B) a terrier mix.

Table 21.4 Levels of consciousness

Level of consciousness	Clinical observation
Alert	Awake, aware, no altered mentation noted
Lethargic	Drowsiness with response to stimuli
Obtunded	Drowsiness with decreased or slow response to stimuli
Stuporous	Only vigorous stimuli will arouse
Comatose	Unresponsive

General nursing care of the neurological patient includes primarily supportive care. Assistance may range from supported walks to chest physiotherapy due to recumbency. Conscious patients permitted to eat yet lack the coordination to do so (i.e., vestibular disease) may require hand feeding as well as help drinking. Some neurological conditions, such as myasthenia gravis, may require the use of lower GI feeding tubes due to esophageal dysfunction.

Assisted walks can be accomplished by using a commercially available (pelvic harness) or by holding a towel or sheet which has been placed under the caudal abdomen to use as a sling. Care should be taken to efficiently provide support, while ensuring that the patient is not overexerted.

Recumbent patients are likely candidates for physical therapy applications. Additionally, if an indwelling urinary catheter is not in place, the bladder should frequently be palpated and expressed. As a general rule, if a patient cannot walk, it is quite possible they cannot urinate efficiently either. Urine retention in the bladder can lead to devastating infections so prevention via bladder maintenance is essential. If a recumbent patient does not have an indwelling urinary catheter in place, consider the benefits for the patients' hygiene and bladder health.

Patients suffering from head trauma or cerebral edema may also benefit from head elevation. A towel or small pillow can be used to obtain elevation. Patients with head trauma should be constantly monitored for level of consciousness (Table 21.4).

As with any patient, measures should be taken to prevent decubital wounds. This holds especially true for the neurological patients who are unable to ambulate on their own. Plenty of padding, foam wedges, and other positional tools should be used to cushion the surfaces under pressure. Frequent positional changes should be implemented as well, changing from right lateral to sternal, left lateral, or semisternal recumbency every 4 hours at least. By implementing positional changes, pressure sores and atelectasis will hopefully not occur.

Chapter references and further reading

C. Dewey (2008) CNS trauma: the first 48 hours. International Veterinary Emergency and Critical Care Symposium.

K. Herzberg (2009) Postoperative nursing care for intervertebral disc disease. *Veterinary Technician the Complete Journal for the Veterinary Hospital Staff* **30**(4): 15-20.

N. Olby (2006) Seizure management: diagnostic and therapeutic principles. *The National Association of Veterinary Technicians in America Journal* **Summer**: 34-39.

J. Osborne, N. Sharp (1998a) Putting "wobblers" back on track–part I. *Veterinary Technician the Complete Journal for the Veterinary Hospital Staff* **19**(7): 449-459.

J. Osborne, N. Sharp (1998b) Putting "wobblers" back on track–part II. *Veterinary Technician the Complete Journal for the Veterinary Hospital Staff* **19**(8): 519-527.

A. Perkinson (2004) Small animal neurologic examination: a practical guide. *Veterinary Technician the Complete Journal for the Veterinary Hospital Staff* **25**(6): 414-424.

S. Platt (2003) Small animal vestibular disease. American Animal Hospital Association Scientific Program.

B. Sturges (2003) Vestibular disease. Western Veterinary Conference.

L. Vaughn (2008) Canine tick paralysis. *Veterinary Technician the Complete Journal for the Veterinary Hospital Staff* **29**(8): 472-477.

Chapter 22
Musculoskeletal Minding

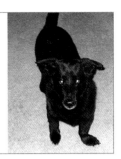

Overview of anatomy and physiology

Approximately 60% of the body is made of muscle. There are three types of muscle: skeletal, which is responsible for movement; smooth (or visceral) muscle; and cardiac muscle. Skeletal muscle is composed of cylindrical, multinucleated fibers which produce movement. Skeletal muscle is striated in appearance due to filaments (actin and myosin) overlapping each other. Actin is a thin filament, whereas myosin is a thick filament, and they attach at cross bridges. The contractual unit of the muscle fiber is the sarcomere; however, muscle contraction requires calcium and energy in the form of adenosine triphosphate (ATP). Skeletal muscle is attached to the bone via tendons (connective tissue; Fig. 22.1).

Motor nerves branch out, innervating many individual muscle fibers, creating a motor unit. The muscle-innervated fibers receive the stimulus and contract simultaneously, enhancing the effect of each individual cell. The terminal ends of each motor neuron are referred to as the neuromuscular junction and contain the neurotransmitter acetylcholine. Acetylcholine is an excitatory neurotransmitter, while acetylcholinesterase works to cease muscle activity by breaking down, or destroying, the acetylcholine. Additionally, energy in the form of ATP is required for contraction as well as calcium ions, which helps activate the contraction. The skeletal muscle uses a sliding mechanism of contraction. In a relaxed state, the actin filaments barely overlap each other. In the contracted state, they slide over each other and are pulled inward among the myosin filaments so they overlap each other almost entirely.

Smooth muscle, or visceral muscle, also uses acetylcholine; however, the physical arrangement of smooth muscle fibers is different from that of skeletal muscle. Smooth muscle requires more calcium ions than skeletal muscle and many smooth muscles require extracellular calcium. Calcium can diffuse to all parts of smooth muscle, allowing contractility. In order to relax the muscle, calcium must be removed out of the smooth

Clinical Small Animal Care: Promoting Patient Health through Preventative Nursing, First Edition.
Kimm Wuestenberg.
© 2012 John Wiley & Sons, Inc. Published 2012 by John Wiley & Sons, Inc.

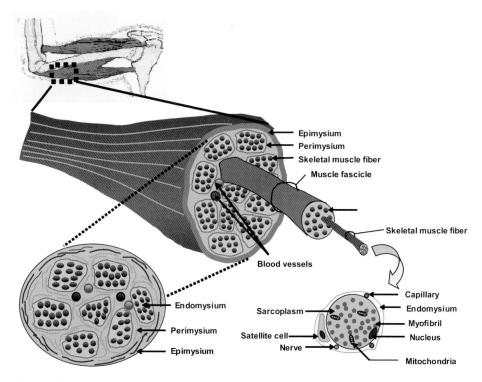

Figure 22.1 Skeletal muscle diagram. Reprinted with permission from Akers, M. and Denbow, M. *Anatomy and Physiology of Domestic Animals*. Wiley-Blackwell, 2008.

muscle fibers. There are no neuromuscular junctions in smooth muscle like there are in skeletal muscle. Nerve fibers instead branch out over muscle fibers and transmit either acetylcholine or norepinephrine to the cells via interstitial fluid. Acetylcholine excites the muscle to contract while norepinephrine inhibits contractions. The terminal axons of smooth muscle have multiple varicosities which hold vesicles containing acetylcholine and norepinephrine (Table 22.1).

Bones have many functions, primarily giving form and rigidity to the body while allowing for movement. They also protect vital organs and support soft tissues. Bones serve as a site for blood formation and a storage area for minerals, particularly calcium and phosphorus. There are two divisions of the skeleton, the axial skeleton and the appendicular skeleton. The axial skeleton consists of the skull, the hyoid apparatus, vertebral column, the costa, and the sternum. The appendicular skeleton is comprised of the limbs. When two or more bones are joined together, a joint is formed. The bones are held by fibrous tissue, elastic tissue, and cartilaginous tissue (Fig. 22.2).

The skeleton is composed of organic bone, which gives elasticity and flexibility, and inorganic bone, which is mainly comprised of calcium and phosphorus at a 1:1 ratio. The formation of bone is called ossification and occurs in two ways: intramembranous and endochondral. Intramembranous growth occurs in flat bones, creating a wider and

Table 22.1 Movement mechanisms

Muscle type	Action
Flexor	Decreases the angle of the joint
Extensor	Increases the angle of the joint
Adductor	Moves limbs toward the median plane
Abductor	Moves limbs away from the median plane
Joint type	**Action**
Plane	Gliding motion in one plane only
Ball and socket	Wide range of motion in many planes
Hinge	Flexion and extension, limited rotation
Pivot	Movement through longitudinal axis
Saddle	Similar to a hinge joint, but with more limited range of motion

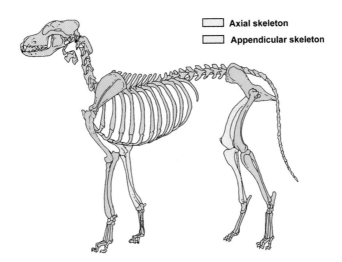

☐ Axial skeleton
☐ Appendicular skeleton

Figure 22.2 The axial and apendicular skeleton. Reprinted with permission from Akers, M. and Denbow, M. *Anatomy and Physiology of Domestic Animals*. Wiley-Blackwell, 2008.

thicker structure. Enchondral growth occurs in long bones, lengthening from the physis or epiphyseal growth plates.

There are two types of structure of bone, compact and cancellous. Compact bone forms the hard, outer layer of bones while cancellous (trabecular or "spongy") bone is found in the middle of flat bones and the ends of long bones and contains bone marrow. The outermost layer of the bone is called the periosteum. The periosteum is comprised of osteoblasts, lymph, blood, and nervous tissue supply and also serves as a point of attachment for ligaments and tendons. Moving further into the bone, the cortical bone is a dense, hard compact bone, which then surrounds the cancellous bone. Within the cancellous bone, there is an epithelial layer, called the endosteum, which is rich in osteoblasts and blood. The medullary canal contains the red and yellow bone marrow. In young animals, the red marrow is wide and contains a large amount of hematopoeitic stem cells. In older animals, the red marrow has been replaced by fat and the canal becomes narrower as blood cell production takes place at the end of long bones (Fig. 22.3).

Bone is rich in blood and nerve supply at the periosteum. There are two major blood supplies to the bone, the nutrient artery and the periosteal vessels. It is through these vessels that blood supply is increased and fracture sites can be stimulated to heal. The nutrient artery is an arterial blood supply to the long bones and the periosteal vessels supply the extremities of the long bones and most of the flat bones. The vessels and

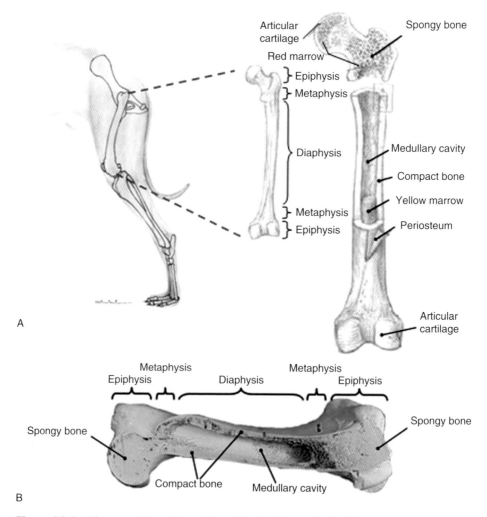

Figure 22.3 Diagram of long bones. Reprinted with permission from Akers, M. and Denbow, M. *Anatomy and Physiology of Domestic Animals*. Wiley-Blackwell, 2008.

Table 22.2   Skeletal structures and functions

Axial skeleton	
Skull	Made up of many small bones which fuse together to form one solid structure. Three divisions: I. Cranium: contains frontal bone, parietal bone, occipital bone, temporal bone, sphenoid bone, and ethmoid bone II. Facial bone: contains palatine, zygomatic, lacrimal, nasal bone, vomer, nasal concha, pterygoid, and the bones containing the teeth III. Middle ear or auditory ossicles: contains malleus, incus, and stapes
Hyoid apparatus	Supports the larynx and the tongue
Vertebral column	Forms the spine, protects the spinal cord, and nerves. There are five divisions: I. Cervical: vertebrae of the neck; dogs and cats have seven cervical vertebrae; the first is referred to as the atlas, the second referred to as the axis II. Thoracic: vertebrae that articulate with a rib; dogs and cats have 13 III. Lumbar: vertebrae of the lower back; dogs and cats have seven IV. Sacral: vertebrae of the sacrum; fused bones which attaches to the pelvis; dogs and cats have three V. Coccygeal: vertebrae of the tail; dogs and cats have 0-24
Costa	Ribs; one pair for each of the thoracic vertebrae. Dorsally bone and ventrally cartilage
Sternum	Flat bone found ventrally at the middle of the chest wall; manubrium is the cranial end and the xiphoid process is the caudal end
Appendicular skeleton	
The forelimb	Scapula, humerus, radius, ulna, carpus, metacarpus, phalanges
The hindlimb	Pelvic girdle (ilium, ischium, pubis, acetabulum), femur, patella, tibia, fibula, flabella, tarsus, metatarsus, phalanges

nerve supply are very important in fracture healing as bone is able to remodel in response to stress applied to it (Table 22.2, Fig. 22.4).

Traumatic muscle injuries

Tendonitis usually occurs with a tear or injury of a tendon, may cause localized pain, inflammation, and swelling. Muscle strains are a tear of the muscle tissue where a muscle is pulled against a force, exceeding the capacity. These muscles are swollen and

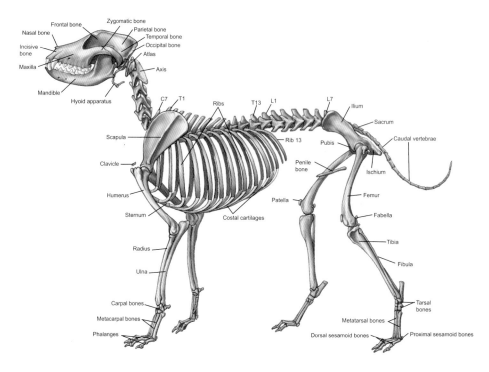

Figure 22.4 The canine skeleton. Reprinted with permission from McCracken, T. and Kainer, R. *Color Atlas of Small Animal Anatomy: The Essentials, Revised Edition.* Wiley-Blackwell, 2009.

painful for the animal. Lacerations, when surgically repaired, generally heal quite well as muscle tissues have a good blood supply.

Infectious muscle disease

Clostridial diseases, primarily tetanus, live in the soil and inhibit nerves, causing contraction of large muscles. Affected muscles usually are the masticatory, triceps, and quadriceps. While the most susceptible hosts are horses and cattle, it may affect dogs and cats. Botulism is the most potent neurotoxin known. The most common cause in humans is from improperly storing canned foods. Botulism causes acute, flaccid paralysis and death usually results from respiratory paralysis. Clinical signs appear within 12–36 hours following ingestion. Toxoplasmosis causes inflammatory myopathy and can occur in any species but is most common in the cat. Neosporum caninum is a recently recognized protozoal disease similar to toxoplasmosis. It is seen in young dogs and may contribute to muscle disease in puppies.

Immune-mediated diseases

Myasthenia gravis occurs when autoantibodies are directed against acetylcholine receptors of the muscle. This leads to profound weakness, paralysis, and paresis.

Esophageal paralysis is a nursing concern as it can lead to food aspiration and subsequent pneumonitis. Masticatory muscle myositis (trigeminal neuritis) is focal, affecting the masseter muscles of the head. Patients will exhibit pain with opening of the mouth. This condition can lead to weight loss since the patient is unable to eat. Polymyositis is a generalized myositis, often associated with systemic lupus erythematosus.

Metabolic disorders affecting muscle

Enzyme deficiencies tend to be rare genetic disorders, but have been reported in Clumber Spaniels. Malignant hyperthermia is relatively rare and usually associated with some older anesthetic agents (halothane and metophane). It occurs when there is a sudden increase in oxygen requirement by striated muscles, causing an increase in lactate production and metabolic acidosis and electrolyte imbalances ensue. Signs of malignant hyperthermia include tachycardia accompanied by arrhythmias leading to bradycardia and cardiac arrest, hyperthermia, muscle rigidity, tachypnea with progression to dyspnea, and finally, apnea. Electrolyte imbalance, particularly calcium and potassium, may cause muscle weakness. Electrolyte imbalances can also have profound effects on the heart and cause arrhythmias. Hyperkalemia can cause bradycardia and lead to asystole while hypokalemia can cause profound weakness. Endocrine disorders such as hypothyroidism, diabetes mellitus, and hyperadrenocortisolism (Cushing's) are also associated with muscle weakness.

Orthopedic

Growth disorders

Osteochondritis dessecans (OCD) is more commonly seen in young, large breed dogs but can also affect cats and small dogs. OCD occurs when a large piece of articular cartilage is poorly attached to the underlying bone. The cartilage piece moves or breaks off into the joint space and causes pain. The shoulder joint is the most commonly affected joint. Canine hip dysplasia (CHD) is a heritable disorder of the formation of the hip joint. The acetabulum and femoral head is flattened, turning the ball and socket joint into a C-shaped joint with a lot of laxity or movement. Elbow dysplasia is a disorder of the formation of the elbow. The most common problem area is an un-united anconeal process, followed by an un-united olecranon process. The elbow joint is extremely intolerant of movement and arthritis will rapidly develop in these joints. Panosteitis, also known as "growing pains," is inflammation of the bone. The cause is unclear but diet has been implicated, leading to the development of large breed-specific diets. The condition is worse when large breed puppies are fed high-protein, high-calorie, and calcium-rich diets. Lameness occurs and these dogs are usually in pain. Signs usually occur at 4-12 months of age and usually the long bones are the affected bones. Premature physeal closure usually results from a compressive or crushing injury to the growth plate. In a complete closure, one leg will be shorter than the other, while a partial closure results with one side of the bone growing longer than the other, causing the bone to curve

Diseases of the bone

Osteomyelitis is an infection of the bone or marrow cavity. There are many causes of osteomyelitis, including (but not limited to) bacterial or fungal infections, open fracture, and other trauma. Neoplastic tumors of bone can be primary bone tumors such as osteosarcoma or secondary (metastatic) tumors associated with cancers such as lymphoma, mammary gland adenocarcinoma, and perianal gland carcinomas. Nutritional disease of the bone is usually a result of vitamin D imbalance or an improper calcium-to-phosphorus ratio in the diet (ratio should be 1:1). Vitamin D is necessary in the uptake of calcium and phosphorus from the gastrointestinal (GI) tract. Osteoporosis is a deficiency of calcium, resulting in thin bone. Osteomalacia is a deficiency in phosphorus, leading to soft bone and otherwise known as "rickets." Metabolic bone disease is an osteomalacia that occurs due to vitamin D deficiency, from either diet, lack of sunlight, or a combination of both (most commonly seen in reptiles).

Diseases of the joints

Degenerative joint disease (DJD) is osteoarthrosis, and commonly known as arthritis. DJD is a painful condition which can develop as a result of trauma, malformation, or age. The joint becomes stiff and loses normal range of motion. Immune-mediated arthritis such as rheumatoid arthritis and systemic lupus erythmatosus occurs when the body's own immune system begins to attack and destroy the articular surfaces of the joints, causing pain and inflammation. Dislocation of the joint is referred to as luxation. It can be complete or partial and can be traumatic or hereditable, such as patellar luxation. Sprains are a trauma to the ligament of a joint, causing instability. In a severe sprain, the ligaments may be completely torn. The carpal joint is the most common joint affected in dogs and cats, most likely due to jumping. Cranial cruciate ligament (CCL) rupture is a very painful condition of the knee in which the ligament becomes torn when the tibia becomes fixed in position and the femur moves forward. Bursitis is an inflammation of the bursa (tendon sheath filled with synovial fluid) of a joint. It usually occurs over a bony protrusion of a joint, with the biceps tendon sheath being the most commonly affected area in dogs.

Miscellaneous orthopedic diseases

Intervertebral disk disease (IVDD) occurs with calcification, rupture, and prolapse (herniation) of the disk material into the vertebral canal. Pressure may be placed on the spinal cord, leading to paralysis or paresis. IVDD is most frequently seen in chondrodystrophic breeds such as the dachshund or Basset Hound, but can affect many breeds of dogs. Spondylosis is a condition where degeneration and bridging of the vertebral bodies occurs. It is extremely common, but in most cases has no significant clinical signs. Cauda equina is a condition of instability and bridging of the lumbosacral (LS) joint. Pain is associated with jumping, and severe cases have fecal and urinary incontinence. Fibrocartilagenous embolism (FCE) occurs when there is a herniation of degenerative disk material into the meningeal or intramedullary blood vessels. FCE can cause acute pain, paresis, or paralysis (Table 22.3).

Table 22.3 Wounds and fractures quick reference

Types of wounds	
Abrasion	The surface of the skin is damaged; however, the damage does not extend to the subdermal layer
Full-thickness defect	The entire layer of skin is missing or torn, revealing the muscle or tissue
Laceration	The skin is cut; usually less damage to the adjacent tissues, but tendons and arteries may suffer trauma
Avulsion	The skin is pulled away from the underlying tissues
Crush	Crushed under pressure or force; associated with the greatest degree of tissue trauma
Wound conditions	
Clean	Surgical wounds; decontaminated then surgically repaired
Clean/contaminated	Relatively clean wounds; less than 6 hours old
Grossly contaminated	Contain debris; require extensive debridement and are more likely to become infected
Infected	Purulent discharge, necrotic tissue; healing cannot occur until the infection is under control
Types of fractures	
Greenstick	Fine, hair-like fracture not completely separated from the shaft
Oblique (spiral)	Break in the shaft that results in two long, sharp points
Transverse	A direct break across the shaft of the bone
Comminuted	A highly fragmented fracture
Salter-Harris	Occurs at the growth plate
Fracture classifications	
Open	Break in the skin; with or without visualization of bone
Closed	No break in the skin

Wounds and fractures

Wounds are classified by the type of wound and the condition of the wound (Fig. 22.5). Wound healing occurs in four stages. Initially, an inflammation stage takes place where various chemical mediators are released. The wound will be red, swollen, warm to the touch, and usually painful. Next, the debridement phase takes place. This a natural cleaning phase involving neutrophils and macrophages. The third phase is repair and re-epithelialization and contraction of the wound. Granulation tissue, which bleeds easily but is resistant to infection, is formed and fills in the wound. Lastly, the maturation phase takes place. This phase may take several years as collagen remodels the wound scar.

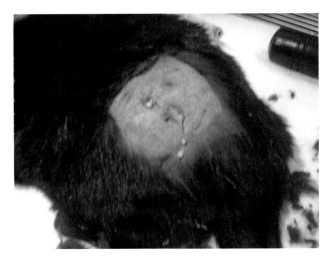

Figure 22.5 Abscess from a cat bite wound.

In addition to the natural healing processes, there are medical management classifications of wound healing. First intention healing is the surgical repair of a wound; second intention healing is where little to no surgical intervention takes place. With second intention healing, wounds take longer to heal and large scars are anticipated. Third intention healing occurs when second intention healing is initiated until enough skin is available to surgically close the wound.

A fracture is a break in the bone. Fractures generally heal well, but slowly. When a bone is fractured, the blood vessels in the area rupture, resulting in hemorrhage. A clot then forms and fibroblasts subsequently form granulation tissue and new capillaries within this clot. Osteoblasts and osteoclasts begin dividing rapidly and a large callus is formed at the end of each bone, eventually bridging the aperture. When the callus becomes fully mineralized, it is remodeled into true bone (this process may take years). A nonunion or improper fracture healing can result in a false joint (pseudarthrosis). This can occur due to a lack of bone-to-bone contact, excessive movement at the fracture site, or in cases of infection, such as osteomyelitis. The main goals in fracture fixation are to immobilize the fracture site, maximize the blood supply, and full return to function while minimizing contamination or infection (Fig. 22.6).

Patients with conditions affecting the musculoskeletal system often need help with positioning and ambulation. Pain management is also warranted, including the application of physical therapy techniques. Patients with bandages should be monitored to ensure perfusion, cleanliness, and comfort. Bandage types, wound dressings, and frequency of changes are generally dependent on the nature of the wound. Bandages that have changed position from original placement or are soiled should be changed. Additionally, patients should be assessed when licking, chewing, biting, or displaying pain associated with the bandage as these are signs of concern (Fig. 22.7-22.9).

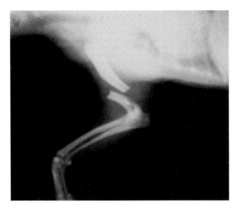

Figure 22.6 Fractured humerus.

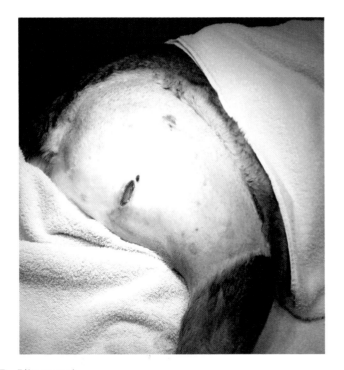

Figure 22.7 Bite wound.

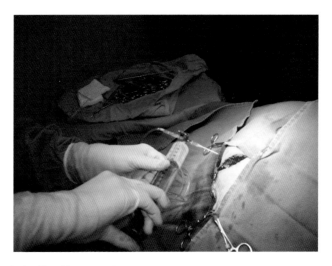

Figure 22.8   Irrigating the wound.

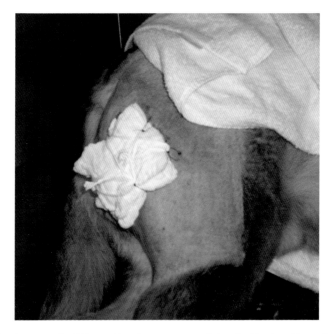

Figure 22.9   A convenient tie-on bandage was used due to the location of wound.

Chapter references and further reading

L. Beagan (2002) Wound healing principles and management. *Veterinary Technician the Complete Journal for the Veterinary Hospital Staff* **23**(11): 667-673.

S. Budsberg (2005) Diagnosis and treatment of osteomyelitis. *The National Association of Veterinary Technicians in America Journal* **Summer**: 45-49.

K. Herzberg (2009) Postoperative nursing care for intervertebral disc disease. *Veterinary Technician the Complete Journal for the Veterinary Hospital Staff* **30**(4): 15-20.

J. Osborne, N. Sharp (1998a) Putting "wobblers" back on track–part I. *Veterinary Technician the Complete Journal for the Veterinary Hospital Staff* **19**(7): 449-459.

J. Osborne, N. Sharp (1998b) Putting "wobblers" back on track–part II. *Veterinary Technician the Complete Journal for the Veterinary Hospital Staff* **19**(8): 519-527.

C. Rhodes (2005) Osteoarthritis in a senior pet. *Veterinary Technician the Complete Journal for the Veterinary Hospital Staff* **26**(10): 702-704.

M. Rhyne (2009) Canine osteoasarcoma. *Veterinary Technician the Complete Journal for the Veterinary Hospital Staff* **30**(12): 12-18.

R. Scalf (2006) Canine traumatic injury. *The National Association of Veterinary Technicians in America Journal* **Winter**: 37-42.

S. Stanley (2007) Impaired wound healing challenges. *The National Association of Veterinary Technicians in America Journal* **Fall**: 39-45.

L. Vaughn (2008) Canine tick paralysis. *Veterinary Technician the Complete Journal for the Veterinary Hospital Staff* **29**(8): 472-477.

Chapter 23

Tending to the Skin and Special Senses

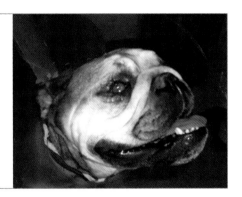

The skin is the largest organ system of the body, making up approximately 6% of body weight. The skin serves as a barrier from the environment, providing protection from physical, chemical, and microbiological injury. The sensory components of the skin enable the perception of heat, cold, pain, touch, and pressure. The skin also functions in vitamin D synthesis and the deeper layers serve as a fat storage depot (Fig. 23.1).

There are three layers: of the skin: the epidermis, the dermis and the subdermis. The epidermis is the avascular outermost layer of the skin. The dermis is of connective tissue origin and contains the epidermal appendages (hair, nails, and the apocrine, eccrine, and sebaceous glands), blood and lymph vessels, and nerves. The subdermis is mostly made up of fat cells but it also contains blood vessels, nerves, and loose connective tissue. The subdermis functions to store fat, preserve body heat, and thermoregulate.

Special senses

The function of the eye is vision. When light passes through the pupil, the lens refracts it to the photoreceptors. The response is then transmitted from the optic nerve to the brain for interpretation. The eyeball, or globe, is made of three layers. The first layer is a fibrous layer consisting of the sclera, which makes up the white part of the eye, and the cornea, which forms the anterior portion of the eye. The cornea is avascular and clear and serves to refract light. The second layer in the globe is the vascular tunic, or uvea. The uvea is comprised of the choroid, which prevents glares; the ciliary body, which serves to help focus; and the iris, which regulates light entering the pupil through contractile action. The ciliary muscles alter the shape of the lens, enabling the eye to focus distance. The iris is the colored portion of the eye and resides between the cornea and the lens. The lens is an avascular clear structure made of protein that focuses light

Clinical Small Animal Care: Promoting Patient Health through Preventative Nursing, First Edition.
Kimm Wuestenberg.
© 2012 John Wiley & Sons, Inc. Published 2012 by John Wiley & Sons, Inc.

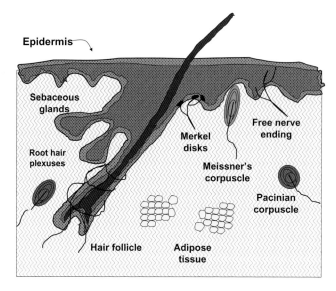

Figure 23.1 Diagram of dermis. Reprinted with permission from Akers, M. and Denbow, M. *Anatomy and Physiology of Domestic Animals*. Wiley-Blackwell, 2008.

onto the last layer of the globe, the retina. Visual images are formed in the retina as it contains the cones and rods, which are photoreceptors. Rods in the retina detect the presence of light, whereas cones detect color.

The globe is separated into three chambers: the anterior, posterior, and vitreous chambers. The anterior chamber is a fluid-filled cavity between the front of the lens and the cornea. The anterior chamber contains the aqueous humor, a fluid that maintains intraocular pressure. The posterior chamber is a fluid-filled cavity between the iris, lens, and ciliary body. Lastly, the vitreous chamber, containing vitreous humor, is located between the iris and the retina. The vitreous humor is a semisolid substance that resides between the retina and the lens (Fig. 23.2).

The eyes have several accessory structures with specific functions. The orbit is formed by the maxilla, zygomatic, frontal, sphenoid, and ethmoid bones. The palpebrae, or eyelids, function to keep the cornea moist, spreading secretions over the globe. Cilia (eyelashes) line the upper and lower eyelids and respond to stimulus with the blink reflex. A thin membrane, the conjunctiva, covers the inside of the eyelids as well as the outer aspect of the globe. The conjunctiva secretes a mucous to keep the globe lubricated. The lacrimal glands, sac, and duct work together in the production and secretion of tears. Tears act to flush debris from the eye and moisten or lubricate. The nictitating membrane ("third eyelid") is a plate of cartilage covered by conjunctiva. It is located medially and moves laterally to cover the eye. It is most notable while patients are ill or under anesthesia. The average dog has a peripheral vision of 120° in each eye, while cats have a peripheral vision of 90° in each eye.

The ear functions in the special sense of hearing. Sound waves transmit through the ear, reach the auditory nerve, and then travel to the brain for interpretation.

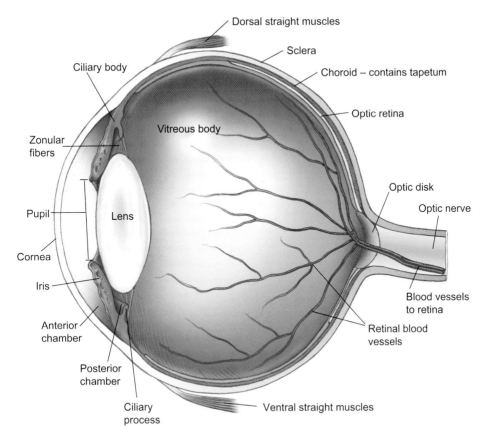

Figure 23.2 Diagram of the eye. Reprinted with permission from McCracken, T. and Kainer, R. *Color Atlas of Small Animal Anatomy: The Essentials, Revised Edition.* Wiley-Blackwell, 2009.

The external ear is made up of the auricle, or pinna, and the external auditory canal. The external auditory canal, or meatus, is the portion of the ear that transmits sound to the middle ear. The middle ear is comprised of the tympanum ("eardrum"); the Eustachian tube, which connects the middle ear to the nasopharynx; and the tympanic bulla. The tympanic bulla is the osseous chamber of the middle ear. It houses three ossicles: the incus, malleus, and stapes. The inner ear contains the vestibule, which aids in balance and equilibrium, and the semicircular canals that contain an area called the ampulla. The ampulla contains sensory cells. Finally, the cochlea, which houses the cochlear duct and organ of Corti, processes sound waves and vibration which send nerve impulses to the brain (Fig. 23.3).

Integumentary system conditions

Pyoderma is an infection of the skin, usually bacterial, fungal, or both. Superficial staphylococcus pyoderma can be primary or secondary with clinical presentation revealing flakes and circular, target-like lesions on the skin, especially the inguinal area.

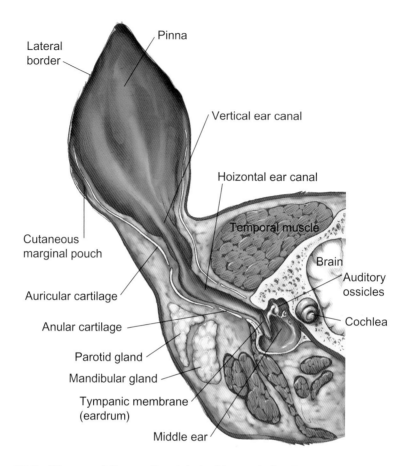

Figure 23.3 Diagram of the ear. Reprinted with permission from McCracken, T. and Kainer, R. *Color Atlas of Small Animal Anatomy: The Essentials, Revised Edition.* Wiley-Blackwell, 2009.

Moist pyoderma, or "hot spot," is most commonly associated with flea bite dermatitis (licking and chewing at affected areas), but can occur in environments where the animal's hair remains moist and warm, such as inadequate drying after a bath or swimming. Skin fold pyoderma is a superficial pyoderma occurring in the skin fold regions of certain breeds such as the Chinese Shar-Pei, pug, Pekingese, and bulldog. Patients with skin folds should have the folds hygienically wiped at least once a day to prevent infection. "Puppy pyoderma" is another superficial staph pyoderma, specifically seen in puppies. The pustules are sterile and not contagious so this is usually controlled with topical shampoos and creams. Deep pyoderma is an infection of the deeper layers of the skin, often extending into the dermis. These animals are usually systemically ill, often requiring oral or injectable antibiotics (Figs. 23.4 and 23.5).

Folliculitis is a variant of staph infection; the bacteria are infecting the hair follicles. It is usually treated with topical management (clip and clean, topical antimicrobial

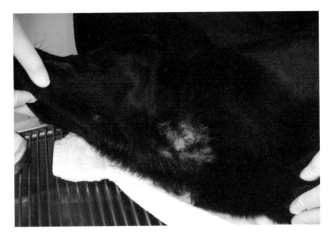

Figure 23.4 Moist pyoderma on the ventral neck of a dog.

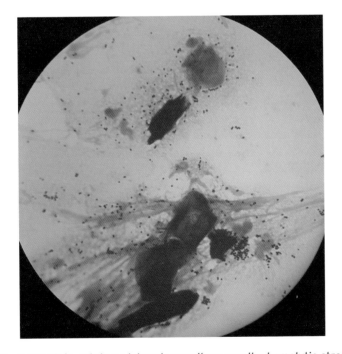

Figure 23.5 Gram stain cytology; laboratory culture results: hemolytic streptococcus.

agents). Feline acne is a folliculitis of the chin in cats. It often begins as comedones (blackheads), which progress to folliculitis.

Malessezia is the most common yeast found in ear canals and skin of the dog and cat. The inner pinna may have a thick, blackened skin, hair loss, a yellow/creamy discharge, and foul odor. Skin and ear cytology will reveal the yeast cells (Fig. 23.6).

Allergic dermatosis is an allergy or hypersensitivity. Atopic dermatitis is an inhalant dermatitis. The pet is allergic to dust, pollen, mites, and so on. When they are inhaled,

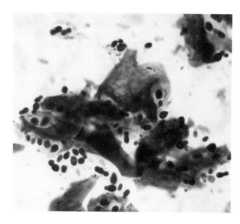

Figure 23.6 Ear cytology: yeast.

the mast cells release histamine in the skin and the pet itches. Flea allergy dermatitis (FAD) is one of the most common skin allergy problems. The animal is allergic to the saliva of the flea. It is important to note that flea allergy is different from flea irritation. Highly allergic animals will scratch intensely for days following a bite.

Food allergy dermatitis is most often caused by meat proteins such as beef, chicken, or lamb, but wheat can also cause problems. Most of these animals also suffer from chronic ear infections and will frequently scratch their face, especially cats. Contact dermatitis is a reaction to an allergen that comes in contact with the skin. Affected areas are common on the ventral abdomen. Carpet powders, detergents, and so on are usually the culprit. Plastic and metal food dishes can also cause contact dermatitis around the lips and muzzle.

Seborrhea is a disorder of the sebaceous gland and keratinization of the skin. It can be a primary or secondary disease. Seborrhea sicca is considered "dry" as the gland does not produce normal amounts of sebum, resulting in dry, flaky skin. Seborrhea oleosa is the "oily" overproduction of the gland, causing waxy, greasy hair coats with layers of greasy scales.

Immune-mediated diseases can affect the integumentary system. Pemphigus can result in hair loss and crusting on the face, muzzle, and ears. Systemic lupus erythematosus (SLE) causes symmetrical skin lesions and usually have other signs associated with the condition such as polyarthritis and kidney disease (Fig. 23.7).

Endocrine diseases that affect the skin are occurring from the inside of the body and displayed on the outside.

Hypothyroidism is commonly seen in the dog, whereas hyperthyroidism is more commonly seen in the cat. Hypothyroid dogs suffer from obesity, dry, brittle hair coats, frequent ear infections, and hair loss with pigmentation on the tail. They may have thickened skin as well. Hyperthyroid cats are often underweight and irritable. They may also have a concurrent renal disease.

Hyperadrenocortisolism, or Cushing's disease, occurs when too much cortisone is produced from the adrenal glands.

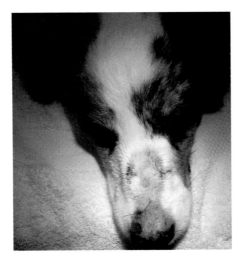

Figure 23.7 Skin biopsy of a dog with pemphigus.

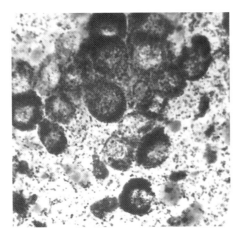

Figure 23.8 Cytology of an MCT.

Neoplasias commonly affecting the skin include squamous cell carcinoma (SCC), malignant melanoma, and mast cell tumors (MCT).

SCC is seen more frequently in cats on ears, nose, and around the eye, and in the oral cavity, particularly sublingual. It begins as "solar dermatitis" with red, scaly areas. It rarely metastasizes but is locally invasive and will recur. Malignant melanoma is usually found in the oral cavity but may be present on the skin. Oral melanoma can be mistaken for pigmented gums; it is important to note that melanoma is brown/black but has rough, uneven edges. MCT are small tumors/nodules on the skin, but can become malignant. These tumors should not be overly palpated as they contain histamine and could release a large amount of histamine and other vasoactive substances (Fig. 23.8).

Other skin conditions include discoid lupus, which is crusting, hair loss, and photosensitivity seen on the bridge of the nose. Zinc deficiency can result in hair loss, thickened gray-white skin, and may be seen in dogs fed a poor quality diet. Psychogenic alopecia occurs when animals lick or chew excessively (neurotically), damaging the skin and hair. An acral lick granuloma is a common behavioral trait in dogs. It may start as an allergic condition, and then the animal licks and chews the spot until it becomes a thickened area of tissue.

Eye (Fig. 23.9)

Common accessory diseases of the eye include conditions such as entropion, ectropion, blepharitis, distichia, conjunctivitis, and follicular ophthalmitis. Entropion occurs when the eyelid rolls inward and rubs on the cornea, causing irritation. Ectropion is the opposite; the eyelid rolls outward, leaving the cornea exposed and dry. Distichia is a condition in which the eyelashes rub on the cornea due to abnormal location. Blepharitis is an inflammation of the eyelids, whereas conjunctivitis is inflammation of the conjunctiva. Conjunctivitis in cats is usually viral (calicivirus, feline viral rhinotracheitis).

Follicular ophthalmitis, otherwise known as "cherry eye," is a condition of hypertrophic and everted nictitating membrane.

Common diseases of the globe include corneal ulceration, keratoconjunctivitis sicca (KCS), cataracts, uveitis, glaucoma, retinal detachment, and proptosis. Corneal ulcers occur when the epithelium of the cornea is interrupted. Ulcers can be caused from a scratch, chemicals (soap), foreign bodies (plant material), or trauma. KCS (or "dry eye") occurs when there is a decrease in production of the watery portion of the tears. This can be medication induced or autoimmune. If treatment is not implemented, these patients will be at risk for corneal ulceration. A cataract is a cloudy lens which may be due to geriatric, heritable, or disease-related causes such as diabetes mellitus. Lenticular sclerosis, however, is the natural aging process of lens hardening, which may be confused with cataract formation. Uveitis is an inflammation of the uvea and usually secondary to a serious disease such as toxoplasmosis, lymphoma, or fungal infections. Glaucoma is a painful condition in which intraocular pressure is increased. Patients with

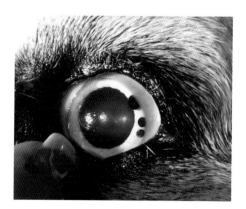

Figure 23.9 Iris cysts.

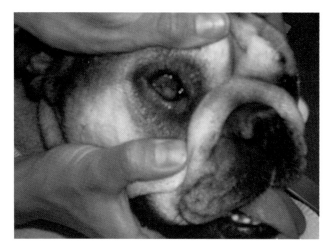

Figure 23.10 Corneal ulcer depicted by fluorescein stain.

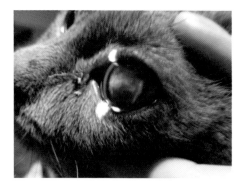

Figure 23.11 Cataract formations in a cat with aqueous misdirection.

glaucoma are at risk for vision loss and should be treated immediately. In acute epi-sodes, a blue haze of the eye may be described by the owner. Additionally, it should be known that patients with glaucoma are at risk for luxating the lens, either into the anterior chamber or posterior chamber (Figs. 23.10 and 23.11).

Proptosis is a traumatic expulsion of the globe from the orbit. These patients should be seen immediately and the expulsed eye lubricated until surgical correction can be performed. Retinal detachment is most notably caused by hypertension and may be seen in patients with renal disease, hyperthyroidism, or other conditions causing sys-temic hypertension. These patients may present with acute blindness, dilated pupils, and a visual retina.

Aural conditions most commonly seen include otitis, aural hematoma, and parasitism. Otitis interna, media, and externa are conditions of inflammation in the inner, middle, and outer ear, respectively. Aural hematomas are often the result of an untreated otitis. Blood vessels in the ear rupture, usually from the pet shaking its head.

Vestibular disease is a neurological disorder that can be caused by an inner ear infec-tion (Figs. 23.12 and 23.13).

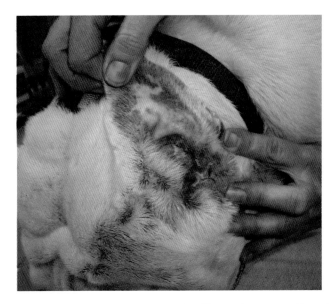

Figure 23.12 Ear infection: cytology revealed bacilli, cocci, mucous threads, and white blood cells (WBCs).

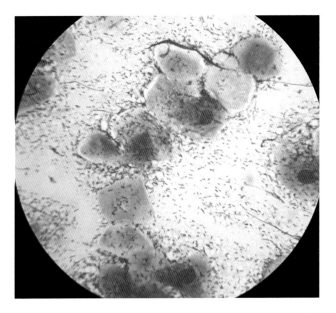

Figure 23.13 Microscopic view of ear cytology; pseudomonas was cultured.

Nursing interventions (Fig. 23.14)

Patients with ocular disease should be thoroughly assessed as systemic disease often manifests through the eyes. Patients should be assessed for vision, pupillary abnormalities, and positional abnormalities. The eyes should be kept clean of debris, moist with lubricant or drops if the patient lacks the ability to close the eye(s). Any patient with eye injury should have an Elizabethan collar in place to prevent further damage (Fig. 23.15, Table 23.1).

The ears should be kept clean and although ear infections may not be a primary disturbance in the patient, the ears should be treated accordingly (Figs. 23.16-23.18).

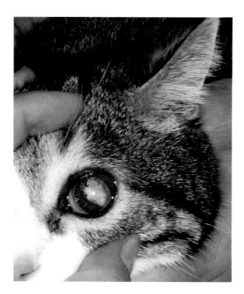

Figure 23.14 Retinal detachment in a panleukopenia survivor.

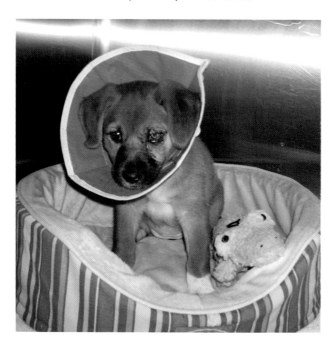

Figure 23.15 An Elizabethan collar placed on a puppy with an eye injury to prevent self-trauma during the healing process.

Table 23.1 Ocular observations

IOP (intraocular pressure): usually decreased in infection and elevated with glaucoma

Schirmer tear test: tests aqueous portion of tear production. Usually decreased in KCS and increased in epiphora.

Fluoroscein stain: tests for corneal lesions. The second layer of the cornea will uptake stain if the surface layer is damaged, leaving the second layer exposed.

PLR (pupillary light reflex): Light response test; tests the integrity of the eyeball and serves as an aid when assessing mental status.

Miotic pupils: small, constricted pupils (light)

Mydriatic pupils: large, dilated pupils (dark)

Anisocoria: Unequal pupil size (Head trauma, feline leukemia virus [FeLV])

Hyphema: blood in the anterior chamber of the eye (trauma)

Strabismus: abnormal pupillary placement; lateral, medial, divergent, or convergent

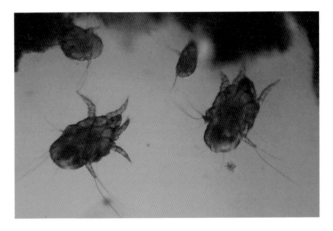

Figure 23.16 Microscopic view of *Otodectes*.

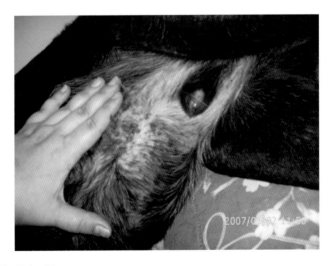

Figure 23.17 Petechiae.

226

The skin should always be kept clean and dry, free of excrement such as urine, feces, vomitus, and saliva. Skin color should be assessed (i.e., jaundice, erythema), as well as examined for the development or changes in bruising patterns (Figs. 23.19 and 23.20).

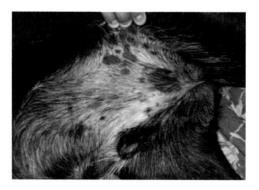

Figure 23.18 Ecchymosis.

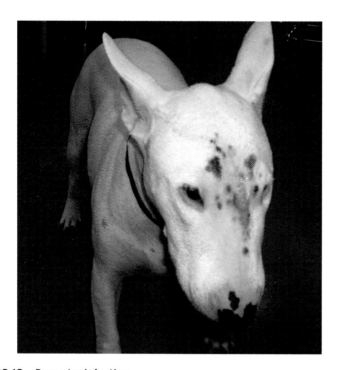

Figure 23.19 *Demodex* infection.

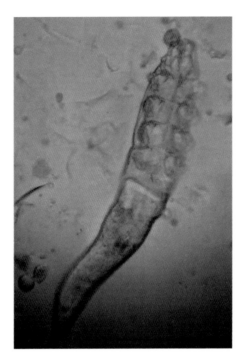

Figure 23.20 Microscopic view of *Demodex*.

Chapter references and further reading

S. Bartelt (2004) The art of tonometry. *Veterinary Technician the Complete Journal for the Veterinary Hospital Staff* **25**(1): 24-26.

P. Basilio (2009) Golden ophthalmic rules. *Veterinary Technician the Complete Journal for the Veterinary Hospital Staff* **30**(10): 21.

L. Beagan (2002) Wound healing principles and management. *Veterinary Technician the Complete Journal for the Veterinary Hospital Staff* **23**(11): 667-673.

M. Berg (2009) Oral pathology. *The National Association of Veterinary Technicians in America Journal* **Winter**: 27-31.

M. Bough (2005) Decontamination procedures. *Veterinary Technician the Complete Journal for the Veterinary Hospital Staff* **26**(8): 548-552.

A. Breton (2005) Deadly dermatological diseases. *The National Association of Veterinary Technicians in America Journal* **Summer**: 38-44.

A. Gordon (2008) Diagnosis of food allergies in dogs and cats. *Veterinary Technician the Complete Journal for the Veterinary Hospital Staff* **29**(6): 350-353.

S. Krick (2003a) Dermatologic disorders and behavior. *Veterinary Technician the Complete Journal for the Veterinary Hospital Staff* **24**(8): 542-546.

S. Krick (2003b) Understanding dermatophytosis. *Veterinary Technician the Complete Journal for the Veterinary Hospital Staff* **24**(8): 514-516.

S. Krick (2004) Understanding glaucoma. *Veterinary Technician the Complete Journal for the Veterinary Hospital Staff* **25**(1): 34-36.

S. Lemarie (2003) Fundamentals of the skin- A cornerstone course. Western Veterinary Conference.

D. Letavish (2004) Ophthalmic examinations: the technician's role. *Veterinary Technician the Complete Journal for the Veterinary Hospital Staff* **25**(1): 10-23.

S. Osborn (2003a) Cutaneous manifestations of systemic disease. Western Veterinary Conference.

S. Osborn (2003b) Management of canine Cushing's disease. Western Veterinary Conference.

S. Osborn (2003c) Review and update for autoimmune skin disease. Western Veterinary Conference.

S. Rhodes (2003) How to handle treating burn injuries. *Veterinary Technician the Complete Journal for the Veterinary Hospital Staff* **24**(6): 392-398.

O. Samples (2005) Basics of ear infections of dogs. *Veterinary Technician the Complete Journal for the Veterinary Hospital Staff* **26**(4): 281-286.

R. Scalf (2006) Canine traumatic injury. *The National Association of Veterinary Technicians in America Journal* **Winter**: 37-42.

B. Stanley (2007) Impaired wound healing challenges. *The National Association of Veterinary Technicians in America Journal* **Fall**: 39-45.

Appendix 1
Formulas

Fluid therapy

Fluid calculations	Formulas
Deficit volume (in mL)	% dehydration × body weight (lb.) × 454 × 0.80
	Or % dehydration × body weight (kg.) × 1000 × 0.80
	Or every 1% increase in packed cell volume (PCV) = 10 mL/kg deficit (using normal values of feline PCV 35% and canine PCV 45%)
Maintenance volume (in mL)	30 × kg + 70 = 24 hours maintenance
	Or 1 mL/lb/h
	Or 50 mL/kg/day (20 mL/kg/day insensible losses, 20 mL/kg/day urine, 10 mL/kg/day feces)
Contemporary losses (vomit/diarrhea)	Milliliters lost × 2

Gravity flow fluid administration calculation

Formula: fluid rate × drip set divided by 360 = drops per 10 seconds
   Example: deliver 40 mL/h using a 20 drops/mL admin set
   Solve: 40 × 20 divided by 360 = 2 drops delivered every 10 seconds
Common administration sets
   10 drops/mL
   15 drops/mL
   20 drops/mL
   60 drops/mL

Clinical Small Animal Care: Promoting Patient Health through Preventative Nursing, First Edition.
Kimm Wuestenberg.
© 2012 John Wiley & Sons, Inc. Published 2012 by John Wiley & Sons, Inc.

Nutrition

Nutritional formulas

Resting energy requirements (RER)	24-hour RER (kcal) = 30 × body weight(kg) + 70 or 60 × body weight(kg) for cats and small dogs
Maintenance energy requirements (MER)	24-hour MER (kcal) = RER × 1.8
Illness energy requirements (IER)	24-hour IER (kcal) = RER × illness factor

Description	Illness factor
Cage rest	1.2
Surgery/trauma	1.3
Multiple surgery/trauma	1.5
Sepsis/neoplasia	1.7
Burns/scalding	2.0
Growth	2.0

Volume of diet to feed	24-hour volume (in milliliters) = IER/energy density (kilocalories per milliliter)

Manual hemogram

Manual hemogram

Value	Procedure	Normal range
Hemoglobin (Hgb) estimate	PCV/3	8-18
Red blood cell (RBC) estimate	PCV/6	5-10
Mean corpuscular volume (MCV)	$\dfrac{PCV \times 10}{RBC}$	40-77
Mean corpuscular hemoglobin (MCH)	$\dfrac{Hgb \times 10}{RBC}$	13-19
Mean corpuscular hemoglobin concentration (MCHC)	$\dfrac{Hgb \times 100}{PCV}$	30-36
Platelet estimate	100× (oil immersion) Use feathered edge of smear Average of 10 fields × 15,000 = platelet count	200,000-900,000

(Continued)

Manual hemogram		
Value	**Procedure**	**Normal range**
White blood cell (WBC) estimate	Observe on 40× Average number of WBCs of 5 fields × 100 and divide by 4	6,000-19,000
WBC differential	Count 100 WBCs on immersion oil (or high dry)	Neutrophils
	Categorize accordingly	Bands: 0%-3%
	Note abnormal morphological features (toxicity quantitation)	Segs: 60%-77%
	Note that a 200 cell count can be used and may be more accurate	Eosinophils: 2%-10%
		Basophils: Rare
		Lymphocytes: 12%-30%
		Monocytes: 3%-10%
RBC morphology	Observe shape, color, size, and arrangement and the presence of parasites	
Reticulocyte count	Stain blood with new methylene blue (NMB) × 10 minutes	<1%
	Prepare blood smear	Regenerative response:
	Observe on 100× (oil immersion)	1%-8% mild
	Calculate % of reticulocytes per 1000 RBCs	9%-15% moderate
	Cats: count aggregate, not punctate	>15% marked

Measurement conversions

Common conversions

1 tbsp.	= 3 tspn.
1 fl oz	= 2 tbsp.
1/4 cup	= 4 tbsp.
1/2 cup	= 8 tbsp.
1 cup	= 8 oz or 240 mL
1 pint	= 2 cups or 16 oz or 480 mL
1 quart	= 4 cups or 2 pints or 960 mL
1 gal	= 4 quarts
1 ft	= 12 in.
1 yard	= 3 ft
1 tspn.	= 5 mL or 60 drops (gtts)
1 tbsp.	= 15 mL
1 oz	= 30 mL
1 g	= 0.035 oz
1 lb	= 454 g
1 kg	= 2.2 lb
1 in.	= 2.54 cm
1 dram	= 4 mL
1 grain	= 64 mg
1 kilocalorie (kcal)	= 1000 calories

Temperature conversion

Centigrade to Fahrenheit	Multiply centigrade number by 9 then divide by 5 and add 32 for Fahrenheit value
Fahrenheit to centigrade	Subtract 32 from the Fahrenheit number, multiply by 5 then divide by 9 for the centigrade value

Body surface conversion

Weight (kg)	Canine (m²)	Weight (kg)	Canine (m²)	Weight (kg)	Feline (m²)	Weight (kg)	Feline (m²)
1	0.101	26	0.886	0.2	0.034	5.2	0.300
2	0.160	27	0.909	0.4	0.054	5.4	0.307
3	0.210	28	0.931	0.6	0.071	5.6	0.315
4	0.255	29	0.953	0.8	0.086	5.8	0.323
5	0.295	30	0.975	1	0.100	6	0.330
6	0.333	31	0.997	1.2	0.113	6.2	0.337
7	0.370	32	1.018	1.4	0.125	6.4	0.345
8	0.404	33	1.029	1.6	0.137	6.6	0.352
9	0.437	34	1.060	1.8	0.148	6.8	0.360
10	0.469	35	1.081	2	0.159	7	0.366
11	0.500	36	1.101	2.2	0.169	7.2	0.373
12	0.529	37	1.121	2.4	0.179	7.4	0.380
13	0.553	38	1.142	2.6	0.189	7.6	0.387
14	0.581	39	1.162	2.8	0.199	7.8	0.393
15	0.608	40	1.181	3	0.208	8	0.400
16	0.641	41	1.201	3.2	0.217	8.2	0.407
17	0.668	42	1.220	3.4	0.226	8.4	0.413
18	0.694	43	1.240	3.6	0.235	8.6	0.420
19	0.719	44	1.259	3.8	0.244	8.8	0.426
20	0.744	45	1.278	4	0.252	9	0.433
21	0.759	46	1.297	4.2	0.260	9.2	0.439
22	0.785	47	1.302	4.4	0.269	9.4	0.445
23	0.817	48	1.334	4.6	0.277	9.6	0.452
24	0.840	49	1.352	4.8	0.285	9.8	0.458
25	0.864	50	1.371	5	0.292	10	0.464

Cytotoxic clearing times

Cytotoxic excretion

Urine

Actinomycin D	Dacarbazine (DTIC)	Cisplatin
Bleomycin	Chlorambucil	Cyclophosphamine
Carboplatin	Melphalan	Methotrexate
		Mitoxantrone

Minimal excretion: doxorubicin, vincristine, vinblastine

Vomit/feces

Actinomycin D	Mitoxantrone	Vinblastine
Doxorubicin	Vincristine	

Minimal excretion: cisplatin, DTIC
Questionable excretion: bleomycin, cyclophosphamine

Estimated clearing time

<1 hour	Bleomycin, cytosine arabinoside, 5-fluorouracil,
2-3 hours	Carboplatin
<12 hours	Chlorambucil, melphalan, methotrexate
24 hours	Vincristine, vinblastine
30-36+ hours	Actinomycin D, doxorubicin, L-asparaginase
<72 hours	Cyclophosphamine
5+ days	Cisplatin, mitoxantrone

Arterial blood gas

Arterial blood gas parameters	Canine	Feline	Unit of measurement
pH	7.35-7.45	7.24-7.45	pH units
PaO_2	80-110	96-118	mmHg
CO_2	35-45	25-37	mmHg
HCO_3	22-27	15-22	mmol/L, mEq/L
Base excess	-2 to +2	-2 to +2.5	mmol/L, mEq/L
SO_2	>90	>90	Percent
Anion gap	12-20	12-18	mEq/L
A-a gradient	10-20	10-20	mmHg

Quick reference chart		
Condition	Primary disturbance	Compensatory factor
Metabolic acidosis	Decreased HCO_3	Decreased $PaCO_2$
Metabolic alkalosis	Increased HCO_3	Increased $PaCO_2$
Respiratory acidosis	Increased $PaCO_2$	Increased HCO_3
Respiratory alkalosis	Decreased $PaCO_2$	Decreased HCO_3

	pH	$PaCO_2$	HCO_3
Fully compensated parameters			
Respiratory acidosis	Normal, but <7.40	Increased	Increased
Respiratory alkalosis	Normal, but >7.40	Decreased	Decreased
Metabolic acidosis	Normal, but <7.40	Decreased	Decreased
Metabolic alkalosis	Normal, but >7.40	Increased	Increased
Partially compensated			
Respiratory acidosis	Decreased	Increased	Increased
Respiratory alkalosis	Increased	Decreased	Decreased
Metabolic acidosis	Decreased	Decreased	Decreased
Metabolic alkalosis	Increased	Increased	Increased

"ROME" mnemonic				
Respiratory				
Opposite				
pH	Increased	$PaCO_2$	Decreased	Alkalosis
pH	Decreased	$PaCO_2$	Increased	Acidosis
Metabolic				
Equal				
pH	Increased	HCO_3	Increased	Alkalosis
pH	Decreased	HCO_3	Decreased	Acidosis

Emergency drug doses

Emergency drug dosing table *(continued on next page)*

Weight #s	Epi (low, 1:1000)	Atropine (0.54 mg/mL)	Vasopressin (20 IU/mL)	Bicarb (8.4%, 1 mEq/mL)	Dopram (20 mg/mL)	Lidocaine (2% (K9), 20 mg/ mL)	Mannitol (20% 20 mg/mL)	Mg chloride (200 mg/ mL)	Naloxone (0.4 mg/ mL)
1	0.05 mL	0.04 mL	0.02 mL	0.5 mL	0.2 mL	0.05 mL	5 mL	10 mL	0.05 mL
5	0.25 mL	0.2 mL	0.1 mL	2.5 mL	1 mL	0.25 mL	25 mL	Over 2 minutes	0.25 mL
10	0.5 mL	0.4 mL	0.2 mL	5 mL	2 mL	0.5 mL	50 mL	⇒	0.5 mL
15	0.75 mL	0.6 mL	0.3 mL	7.5 mL	3 mL	0.75 mL	75 mL		0.75 mL
20	1 mL	0.8 mL	0.4 mL	10 mL	4 mL	1 mL	100 mL		1 mL
25	1.25 mL	1 mL	0.7 mL	12.5 mL	5 mL	1.25 mL	125 mL		1.25 mL
30	1.5 mL	1.2 mL	0.8 mL	15 mL	6 mL	1.5 mL	150 mL		1.5 mL
35	1.75 mL	1.4 mL	0.9 mL	17.5 mL	7 mL	1.75 mL	175 mL		1.75 mL
40	2 mL	1.6 mL	1 mL	20 mL	8 mL	2 mL	200 mL		2 mL
45	2.25 mL	1.8 mL	1.1 mL	22.5 mL	9 mL	2.25 mL	225 mL		2.25 mL
50	2.50 mL	2 mL	1.2 mL	25 mL	10 mL	2.5 mL	250 mL		2.5 mL
55	2.75 mL	2.2 mL	1.3 mL	27.5 mL	11 mL	2.75 mL	275 mL		2.75 mL
60	3 mL	2.4 mL	1.4 mL	30 mL	12 mL	3 mL	300 mL		3 mL
65	3.25 mL	2.6 mL	1.7 mL	32.5 mL	13 mL	3.25 mL	325 mL		3.25 mL
70	3.5 mL	3 mL	1.8 mL	35 mL	14 mL	3.5 mL	350 mL		3.5 mL
75	3.75 mL	3.2 mL	1.9 mL	37.5 mL	15 mL	3.75 mL	375 mL		3.75 mL
80	4 mL	3.4 mL	2 mL	40 mL	16 mL	4 mL	400 mL		4 mL
85	4.25 mL	3.6 mL	2.1 mL	42.5 mL	17 mL	4.25 mL	425 mL		4.25 mL
90	4.5 mL	4 mL	2.2 mL	45 mL	18 mL	4.5 mL	450 mL		4.5 mL
95	4.75 mL	4.2 mL	2.3 mL	47.5 mL	19 mL	4.75 mL	475 mL		4.75 mL
100	5 mL	4.4 mL	2.4 mL	50 mL	20 mL	5 mL	500 mL		5 mL
Dose	0.1 mg/kg double for intratracheal (IT)	0.05 mg/kg	0.8 IU/kg	1 mEq/kg over 10 minute	2 mg/kg	2 mg/kg; 0.5 mg/kg fel	0.5 g/kg over 20–30 minute	2 g over 2 minute	0.4 mg/ kg

Appendix 2
Anatomy Illustrations

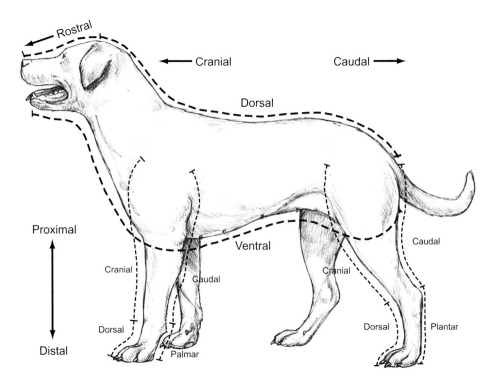

Figure A1 Positional and directional terms. Reprinted with permission from McCracken, T. and Kainer, R. *Color Atlas of Small Animal Anatomy: The Essentials, Revised Edition.* Wiley-Blackwell, 2009.

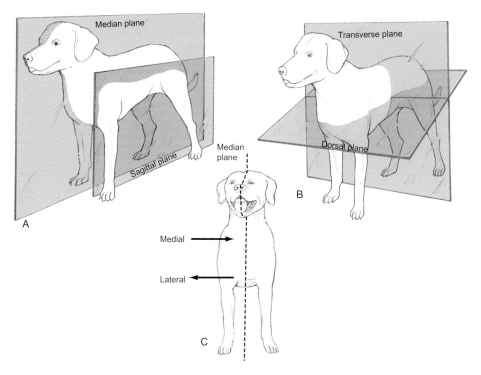

Figure A2 Body planes. Reprinted with permission from McCracken, T. and Kainer, R. *Color Atlas of Small Animal Anatomy: The Essentials, Revised Edition.* Wiley-Blackwell, 2009.

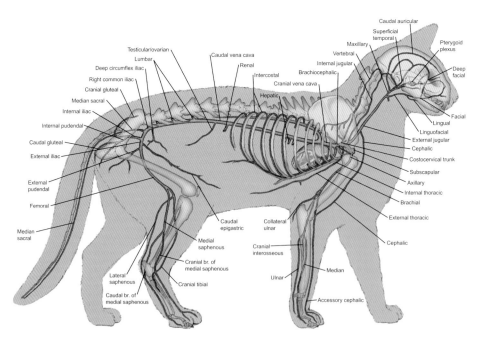

Figure A3 Major veins in felines. Reprinted with permission from McCracken, T. and Kainer, R. *Color Atlas of Small Animal Anatomy: The Essentials, Revised Edition.* Wiley-Blackwell, 2009.

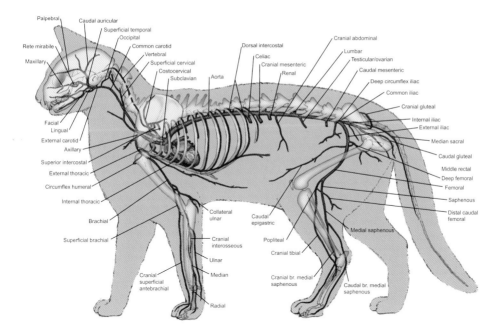

Figure A4 Major arteries in felines. Reprinted with permission from McCracken, T. and Kainer, R. *Color Atlas of Small Animal Anatomy: The Essentials, Revised Edition.* Wiley-Blackwell, 2009.

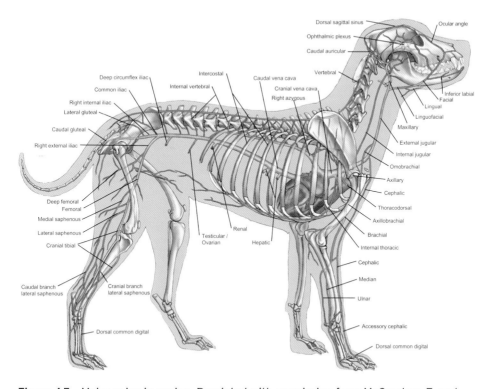

Figure A5 Major veins in canine. Reprinted with permission from McCracken, T. and Kainer, R. *Color Atlas of Small Animal Anatomy: The Essentials, Revised Edition.* Wiley-Blackwell, 2009.

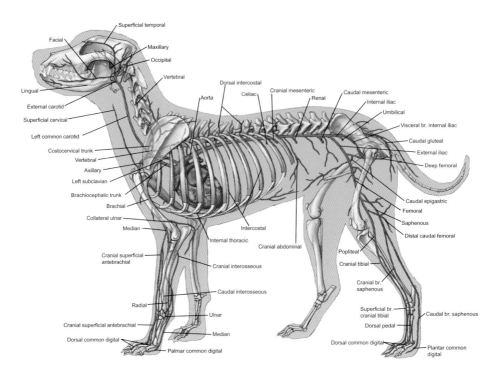

Figure A6   Major arteries in canines. Reprinted with permission from McCracken, T. and Kainer, R. *Color Atlas of Small Animal Anatomy: The Essentials, Revised Edition.* Wiley-Blackwell, 2009.

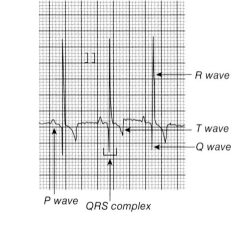

A

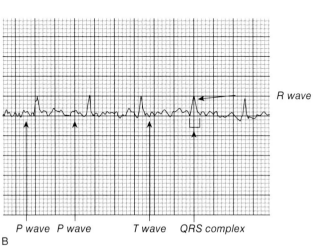

B

Figure A7 Heart excitation and electrocardiograph (ECG) tracing. Reprinted with permission from Akers, M. and Denbow, M. *Anatomy and Physiology of Domestic Animals*. Wiley-Blackwell, 2008.

Appendix 3
Clinical Quick Reference Guides

Abbreviations

Prescriptions		Exam	
Rx	To take	Hx	History
SID	Once a day	PE	Physical exam
BID	Twice a day	SOAP	Subjective, objective, assessment, plan
TID	Three times a day	TPR	Temp, pulse, respiration
QID	Four times a day	HR	Heart rate
qd, q24h	Once daily	RR	Respiratory rate
QOD, eod	Every other day	MM	Mucous membranes
prn	As needed	CRT	Capillary refill time
a.c.	before meals, ante cibum	WT	Weight
p.c.	after meals, post cibum	kg	Kilograms
po, per os	By mouth	lb.	Pounds
NPO	Nothing by mouth	g	Grams
AS	Left ear	m^2	Meters squared
AD	Right ear	QAR	Quiet, alert, responsive

(Continued)

Clinical Small Animal Care: Promoting Patient Health through Preventative Nursing, First Edition.
Kimm Wuestenberg.
© 2012 John Wiley & Sons, Inc. Published 2012 by John Wiley & Sons, Inc.

(Continued)

Prescriptions		Exam	
AU	Both ears	BAR	Bright, alert, responsive
OS	Left eye	p/u	Polyuric
OD	Right eye	p/p	Polyphagic
OU	Both eyes	p/d	Polydipsic
Gtt, gtts	Drop, drops	e/d/u/d	Eating, drinking, urinating, defecating
cap	Capsule	c-s	Coughing, sneezing
tab	Tablet	v/d	Vomiting, diarrhea
sol	Solution	BM	Bowel movement
oint	Ointment	u/o	Urine output
pwd	Powder	r/o	Rule out
bol	Bolus	ENT	Ears, nose, throat
ss	One-half	EENT	Eyes, ears, nose, throat
s	One	Dx	Diagnosis
OTC	Over the counter	DDx	Differential diagnosis
BBB	Blood–brain barrier	Px	Prognosis
TD	Transdermal	WNL	Within normal limits
IM	Intramuscular	RTG	Ready to go
SQ, SC	Subcutaneous	PT	Physical therapy
ID	Intradermal	CPT	Chest physiotherapy
IP	Intraperitoneal	P&A	Percussion and auscultation
IT	Intratracheal	ML	Midline
IA	Intra-arterial	TLC	Tender loving care

Vital signs

Parameter	Feline	Canine
Heart rate (HR)	160–220 beats per minute (bpm)	100–160 bpm (small breed) 60–100 bpm (large breed)
Respiratory rate (RR)	20–30 breaths per minute	10–30 breaths per minute
Temperature	100.5–102.5°F	100.2–102.8°F
Blood pressure	120/80; mean arterial pressure (MAP) 80–90 mmHg	120/80; MAP 80–90 mmHg

Emergency assessment

Triage: airway, breathing, circulation (ABCs)

Supportive care

Fluid balance

Blood pressure

Perfusion

Heart rate and rhythm

Pulse quality and synchronicity

Oxygenation and ventilation

Database: packed cell volume/total solids (PCV/TS), blood glucose (BG), arterial blood gas (ABG), electrolytes

Mentation

Body systems review

Pain management

Stages of shock

Physical parameters	Compensatory stage (early phase)	Decompensatory stage (middle phase)	Terminal stage (end phase)
Heart rate	Normal to mild elevation	Tachycardia	Severe bradycardia
Pulse quality	Normal to bounding	Poor	Absent
Blood pressure	Normal	Hypotension	Severe hypotension
Respiratory rate	Eupneic or mild elevation	Tachypneia	Bradypnea or apnea
Mucous membrane (MM)	Normal to injected	Pallor	Pallor
Capillary refill time (CRT)	<1 second	>2 seconds	>5 seconds or absent
Temperature	Euthermic or slightly elevated	Hypothermia	Profound hypothermia
Mentation	Normal, alert, or excited	Depressed or obtunded	Stuperous or comatose
Physiological effects of shock	Neurohormonal (neuroendocrine) response, hypermetabolic	Shunting of blood to vital organs, O_2 consumption dependent on O_2 delivery, metabolic acidosis	Dysfunctional blood flow *circulus vitiosis*, impending cardiopulmonary arrest (CPA)

Types of shock

Types of Shock	Cause	Examples
Hypovolemic	Low blood volume	Anemia, hemorrhage
Neurogenic	Nervous system effect	Toxins such as ethylene glycol or strychnine
Cardiogenic	Heart disease	Congestive heart failure (CHF), pericardial tamponade
Anaphylactic	Massive immune response	Bee sting, vaccination
Septic	Bacteria endotoxin	Sepsis

Electrolyte disorders

Electrolyte disorders	Potential causes
Hypokalemia	Dilutional, alkalosis, gastrointestinal (GI) loss, renal loss
Hyperkalemia	Urinary tract obstruction (UTO), hypoadrenalcorticism, Addisonian crisis
Hypocalcemia	Hypoparathyroidism, hypoproteinemia, vitamin D deficiency, hyperphosphatemia, malabsorption, acute pancreatitis, chronic renal disease, eclampsia
Hypercalcemia	Pseudohyperparathyroidism, primary hyperparathyroidism, cholecalciferol-containing rodenticides
Hyponatremia	Water excess or salt loss
Hypernatremia	Water loss or salt gain

Anesthesia (Ax) monitoring and troubleshooting

Setup

- Assess oxygen supply
- Test Ax machine for leaks
- Double-, triple-check all attachments on machine
- Verify CO_2 adsorbent is not exhausted
- Examine the Ax patient
- Be familiar with conditions/diseases and signalment
- Be familiar with the mode of action and side effects of Ax agents used
  - Hydromorphone/morphine may cause vomiting
  - Buprenorphine may cause low body temperature
  - Acepromazine may cause low blood pressure
  - Propofol may cause apnea
  - Some opiates can result in a mild hyperthermia, especially in cats
  - Medetomadine causes a slow heart rate due to core shunting
- Be familiar with the surgery (Sx)/Ax procedure and anticipate responses
  - Neuters: May become light with testicular pulling
  - Spays: May become light with ligament, ovarian, or uterine horn pressure/handling
  - Dentals: May become light during extractions, probing, and even scaling and polishing
  - Hypothermia: Particularly in small patients, open chest/abdomen, or long procedures

Multiparameter monitoring

- YOU are the BEST monitor!
  - Physical assessment of respiratory rate and pattern
  - Physical assessment of heart sounds and pulse quality
- Electrocardiography (ECG)
  - Heart rate and rhythm
- Capnograph
  - Respiratory rate and gas exchange
- Pulse oximetry
  - Oxygen saturation of hemoglobin
  - Oxygen detected in that vessel only!
- Blood pressure
  - Systemic perfusion!
  - Must remain above 60 mmHg
  - If blood is flowing to the tissues → hypoxia → cell death
- Temperature
  - Patients kept warm recover smoother
  - Less chance of infection
  - Less painful
- Constant assessment
  - Heart rate and pulse rate/quality
  - Respiratory rate and pattern
  - Body temperature
  - Ax depth: under enough to not feel pain, but not so deep they become compromised

Transfusions

Anemias	Cause	Examples
Regenerative	Parasitism blood loss	
	Internal	Hookworm
	External	Flea, louse, tick
	Excessive red blood cell (RBC) destruction	
	Extracorpuscular	Immune-mediated hemolytic anemia
		Intravascular fragmentation
	Intracorpuscular	Lead poisoning
		Pyruvate kinase deficiency
Nonregenerative	Nutritional	Deficiency in iron, copper
	Bone marrow failure	RBC aplasia
		Aplastic anemia
	Anemia of chronic disease	Renal, hepatic, neoplastic

Hemostatic disorders		
Coagulation protein disorders	Congenital	Factor I: Congenital afibrinogenemia
		Factor II: Prothrombin disorders
		Factor VIII: Hemophelia A
		Factor IX: Hemophelia B
	Acquired	Anticoagulant rodenticide ingestion
		Disseminated Intravascular Coagulation
Thrombocytopenia	Congenital	Cyclic hematopoiesis in gray Collie dogs
	Acquired	*Ehrlichia*
		Primary immune mediated Thrombocytopenia
		Vaccine-induced thrombocytopenia
		Drug-induced thrombocytopenia
Platelet dysfunction	Congenital (intrinsic)	Chediak–Higashi syndrome
		Canine thrombopathia
	Congenital (extrinsic)	Von Willebrand disease
	Acquired	Immune-mediated thrombocytopenia
		May occur secondary to systemic or infectious disease
		Drugs inhibiting platelet response
Pathological thrombosis	Primary or inherited anticoagulant disorders	
	Secondary or acquired anticoagulant disorders	

Simple 10-step blood cross-match

1. Centrifuge donor and recipient ethylenediaminetetraacetic acid (EDTA) blood (lavender top tube, LTT) for 10 minutes
2. Label two plain red top tubes "Donor" and "Recipient"
3. Remove plasma from tubes and place accordingly
4. Remove 0.2 mL of RBCs from EDTA and tube
5. Place in 4.8 mL of normal saline
6. Mix gently
7. Label three separate plain red top tubes: "Major," "Minor," and "Control"
8. Prepare accordingly:
   Major: Add 0.1 mL of Donor RBC solution and 0.1 mL Recipient plasma
   Minor: Add 0.1 mL of Donor plasma and 0.1 mL Recipient RBC solution
   Control: Add 0.1 mL of Recipient plasma and 0.1 mL Recipient RBC solution
9. Incubate at room temperature for 15 minutes
10. Examine all samples grossly and microscopically for hemolysis or agglutination

Blood product transfusion reference

Fresh whole blood	Collected immediately prior to transfusion
	Viable platelets, RBCs, white blood cells (WBCs), all clotting factors, and plasma proteins
Stored whole blood	RBCs, WBCs, plasma proteins
	Platelets viable for 2 hours
	Clotting factors (V, VIII) viable for 24 hours
pRBCs	RBCs separated from plasma
Fresh frozen plasma (FFP)	Plasma separated from fresh whole blood
	Frozen within 6-8 hours of collection
	Contains all clotting factors, including factors V and VIII
Frozen (stored) plasma (FP)	Separation of plasma and RBCs after centrifugation (at any time)
	Prepared >6-8 hours after blood collection = small amounts of factors V and VIII
	Does contain all vitamin K-dependent factors = effective in the treatment of warfarin toxicity
	Contains plasma proteins
Cryoprecipitate	Prepared from FFP
	Concentration 10-fold less than FFP of clotting factor VIII, von Willebrand factor, and fibrinogen
	Contains clotting factors XI and XIII and fibronectin
Immune reactions	Acute hemolysis · Delayed hemolysis
	Fever · Anaphylaxis

(Continued)

(Continued)

Blood product transfusion reference

Nonimmune reactions	Septicemia	Air embolism	Circulatory overload
	Hypercalcemia	Hemorrhagic diathesis	Transmission of disease
	Septicemia		
Packed red blood cells (PRBC) or whole blood artifacts	Irregular clumps of white or off-white material or layers floating on top		WBCs and platelet aggregates: use filter
	Regular, entire white bodies		Possible bacteria colonies: do not use
	White flecks resembling paint chips		Fat -will dissolve into solution as the unit is warmed.
	Visible hemolysis in the segments or unit		Outdated or contaminated with bacteria: do not use
FFP artifacts	White stringy material		Precipitated coagulation factor VIII and fibrinogen: use filter
	Milky white in color when thawed		Fat
	Regular, entire white bodies		Possible bacteria colonies: do not use

Pearls of wisdom

Pearls of wisdom	
Mucous membrane assessment	
Pallor	Hypoxia, shock, anemia, epinephrine injection
Yellow hue	Anemic pallor plus icterus
Orange hue	Pink mucous membranes plus icterus
Gastrointestinal	
Bile in vomitus	Signifies pyloric patency
Coffee ground vomitus	Gastric ulcers, uremic gastritis
The more feculent the vomitus	The lower the obstruction
Melena or black stools	Upper GI bleed/lesion, thrombocytopenia, swallowing blood, iron, charcoal
Frank red stool	Large bowel
Urogenital	
Bilirubinuria in cats	Suggests liver disease
Glycosuria	Can occur with diabetes, proximal renal tubular disease, stress, intravenous (IV) dextrose
Marked hyperglycemia with minimal glycosuria	Consider oliguria/anuria
Milky urine	Pus, chyle, crystals
Cardiorespiratory	
Muffled chest sounds	Fluid, mass, air, obesity, deep chested
Diffuse muffling	Usually chest fluid
Dorsal muffling	Air or mass in chest
Coughing cat	Allergic bronchitis, flukes, lung worms, heartworms, hair in trachea. Cats with heart disease rarely cough
Acute respiratory distress syndrome (ARDS)	Sudden onset diffuse pulmonary infiltrates
Hyperventilation	Cardiorespiratory, pyrexia, brain disease, Cushing's, metabolic acidosis, anxiety, pain, shock, anemia

(Continued)

(Continued)

Pearls of wisdom	
X-ray	Good side UP, Oxygen available
Coagulation	
Clot tube doesn't clot	Consider coagulopathy
Pale petechia	Thrombocytopenia plus anemia
Lumbosacral petechia	Fleas plus thrombocytopenia
Normal bleeding time	Ensures adequate platelet hemostasis
Normal platelet count	Does not ensure adequate platelet hemostasis
Neuro	
Traumatic ear flush	Can lead to vestibular disease
Rapid onset lower motor neuron (LMN) paralysis	Ticks, organophosphate, botulism, polyradiculoneuropathy, metronidazole, coral snake
Oliguric renal failure	Hyperkalemia
High output chronic renal failure	Normal potassium level or hypokalemia
General	
Clean patient	Happy patient
Body bandage in cats	Causes pseudoparalysis
Urine specific gravity (USG)	Prior to fluid therapy
Fever	Plus immune-mediated disease–appetite can persist
	Plus sepsis–anorexia
Early signs of weakness	Hind legs
Skin turgor	Difficult to assess with cachexia and obesity
Diabetic order	BG level, feed, insulin
Diabetes mellitus	Increased USG
Diabetes insipidus	Decreased USG

Source: Schaer, M. Clinical pearls in intensive and critical care I & II (VET-78, VET-79). New Jersey Veterinary Medical Association Annual Meeting, 2010.

Appendix 4
General Forms

Sample treatment flow sheet

Patient	
Client	
Phone #	
Date	

Weight	lb.	kg
Diagnosis		
Fluid Type/Rate		
Caloric Requirements		

	8AM	10AM	12PM	2PM	4PM	6PM	8PM	10PM	12AM	2AM	4AM	6AM
Fluid Total												
Temp												
HR/Pulse Quality												
RR/Pattern												
Mentation												
Walk												
u/o												
BM												
Diet _____												
Calories In												
Medications:												
1)												
2)												
3)												
4)												
5)												
Other:												
Notes on Back	1	2	3	4	5	6	7	8	9	10	11	12

Clinical Small Animal Care: Promoting Patient Health through Preventative Nursing, First Edition.
Kimm Wuestenberg.
© 2012 John Wiley & Sons, Inc. Published 2012 by John Wiley & Sons, Inc.

Daily Care

Flush IVC	
Strip Down and Rewrap IVC	
Clean Kennel, Fresh Bedding	
Maintain Hygiene	
Calculate Ins/Outs	

Additional Treatments every _____ hours

BP		ECG		U. Cath Care	
Oxygen		PLR		Central Line Care	
Rotate		Heat/Ice		IO Cath Care	
PROM		Massage		Chest Tube Care	
Nebulize		Coupage		Feeding Tube Care	

	Initials	Notes
1		
2		
3		
4		
5		
6		
7		
8		
9		
10		
11		
12		

ICU monitoring flow sheet

Date:		Patient:			Owner:		Tech:
Condition:					Dr:		

Meds	Strength	Dose	Route	Time	Initials	DNR:		Wt:
						IVC		
						Special Concerns:		
							Fluid Type:	
							Rate:	
							Total Volume:	
						Monitoring:		
						Pulse Ox ☐	Bp ☐	
						ECG ☐	Temp ☐	
						Capnograph ☐	Other: ☐	

Time:										
Fluids In										
Fluids Out										
O$_2$ Rate										
Pulse Ox:										
Temp:										
190										
180										
170										
160										
150										
140										
130										
120										
110										
100										
90										
80										
70										
60										
50										
40										
30										
20										
10										
0										

HR ●	Notes:
RR ○	
Sys ⌂	
Dias ♥	
MAP ☆	

Anesthetic record

Date:	Patient:	Owner:	Risk Factor: 1 2 3 4 5

Procedure:	Dr:	Tech:

PreAx Med	Strength	Dose	Route	Time	Initials

Time:	Temp:	Wt:
HR:	RR:	MM:
IVC		Ax Type:

Special Concerns:

Induction	Dose	Amt Given	Route	Time
Chamber	Mask	ET Tube Size:		

Fluid Type:
Rate:
Total Volume:

Intra-Op	Strength	Dose	Route	Time	Initials

Monitoring:

Pulse Ox	☐	BP	☐
ECG	☐	Temp	☐
Capnograph	☐	Other:	☐

Ax Start:		Ax End:	
Sx Start:		Sx End:	
Extubated:			

Time:									
Ax Rate:									
O$_2$ Rate									
Pulse Ox:									
ETCO$_2$									
Temp:									
190									
180									
170									
160									
150									
140									
130									
120									
110									
100									
90									
80									
70									
60									
50									
40									
30									
20									
10									
0									

HR ●	Notes:			Post-Op	Time	HR	RR	Temp
RR ○								
Sys ⌂								
Dias ♡								
MAP ☆								

Patient order sheet

Patient_____ Owner _____ Date_____

Fluids
IVC → Bolus_____ Rate_____ SQ Fuids → Amount_____
Fluid Type: LRS   Norm-R   0.9%NaCl   Other_____
Fluid Additives Vitamin B_____ KCl_____ Dextrose _____
                   Other_____

Blood Collection
In-House → PCV/TS Glucose CBC Chemistries Coags
Other_____
Urine Collection → Free Catch Catheter Cystocentesis
In-House U/A Chemistry Only USG Only Sediment Only C/S
Other_____

Ancillary Testing
ECG BP Pulse Oximetry Radiographs U/S

Meds

ROUTE	Medication and Concentration	Amount (mg/mL)
PO SQ IM IV		
PO SQ IM IV		
PO SQ IM IV		
PO SQ IM IV		
PO SQ IM IV		

Nutrition
NPO   Special Diet _____ Feed q _____ hours
Other:

_____
_____
_____

Case transfer form for opposing shifts

Date_____ Dr._____ Primary Technician(s)_____

Pet Name_____ Owner_____ Client #_____

Signalment_____ Diagnosis/Reason for Treatment_____

Treatments (Tx) Needed As Follows:

Time	Tx	Completed (Initial)

ABC animal hospital

Client communication log

☐ **Dr. A**   ☐ **Dr. B**   ☐ **Dr. C**

Patient:	Owner:	Client #:	Date:

Laboratory Results:
- ☐ Normal
- ☐ Abnormal
  - Comment:
- ☐ OK for Ax
- ☐ Recheck Labs
  - ____days
  - ____weeks
  - ____months
- ☐ Other:

Prescriptions:
- ☐ New Medication
- ☐ Medication Change
- ☐ Due for Lab Work
- ☐ Needs Exam Before Next Refill
- ☐ Needs Exam Before This Refill
- ☐ Other:

Referral Needed:
- ☐ Surgical
- ☐ Internal Medicine
- ☐ Dermatology
- ☐ Ophthalmology
- ☐ Dentistry
- ☐ Technician Arranged Appointment

Miscellaneous:
- ☐ Appointment Needed
  - ⇨Exam
  - ⇨Recheck
  - ⇨Consult
  - ⇨Telephone Follow-Up with Tech
  - ⇨Other
- ☐ Diet/Nutrition
- ☐ Physical Therapy
- ☐ Diagnostics
  - ⇨Lab Work (In-House)
  - ⇨Lab Work (Outside Lab)
  - ⇨Urine via Cystocentesis
  - ⇨Urine Drop Off
  - ⇨Fecal Drop Off
  - ⇨HW Test Due
  - ⇨Cytology
  - ⇨Radiograph
  - ⇨Ultrasound (In-House)
  - ⇨ECG
  - ⇨Tonometry
  - ⇨Blood Pressure (Doppler)
- ☐ Other:
- ☐ Notes:

Owner Notified

Date:	Time:	Technician Initials:		

- ☐ Talked Directly to Owner
- ☐ Left Message on Answering Machine/Voicemail
- ☐ Unable to Reach Owner–3 Attempts:

Date/Time	Date/Time	Date/Time

- ☐ Comments:

Appendix 5

Employee Skill and Knowledge Advancement Plans

Assistant level skills mastery form

General nursing

Skill to be mastered	Completed	Date	Supervisor
Basic medical terminology			
Canine restraint			
Feline restraint			
Knowledge of normal vital signs			
Obtain vital signs			
Obtain history from client			
Assist DVM in exam room			
Vaccination knowledge and understanding			
Heartworm disease knowledge and understanding			
Benefits of o/c and ovh			
Dental care/health			
Importance of fecal testing (parasites)			
TNT			
Ear clean			
Anal gland expressing (internal and external)			

Clinical Small Animal Care: Promoting Patient Health through Preventative Nursing, First Edition. Kimm Wuestenberg.
© 2012 John Wiley & Sons, Inc. Published 2012 by John Wiley & Sons, Inc.

Pharmacology skills

Knowledge of drug classifications

Pharmacology terminology

Prepare prescriptions

Log control substances

Perform drug calculations
(have a tech check)

Administer oral medications

Administer SQ injections

Apply topical medications

Instill ear medications

Instill eye medications
Medicated bathing

Laboratory skills

Properly log lab samples

Prepare requisition form

Prepare cytology samples

Proper handling of specimens
(urine, tissue, serum, etc.)

Perform urine chemistry and USG

Perform PCV/TS

Make a blood smear

Perform HWT (4dx)

Perform FeLV/FIV test

Perform CpL test

Perform Giardia snap test

Perform Parvo test

Prepare direct fecal

Prepare fecal floatation

Use in-house laboratory machines

Prepare Bartonella test

Radiology skills

Properly measure for radiographs

Properly perform radiographs (positioning)

Develop radiographs

Label and file radiographs

Dental radiograph developing (manual)

Knowledge of digital radiographs/
radiograph program

Properly use PPE

Understand radiograph anatomy

Perform Barium series

Anesthesia skills

Basic understanding of Ax effects on patient

Basic understanding of multiparameter
monitoring

Familiarity with types of Ax

Understanding of Ax machine

Ax machine testing

Ax machine troubleshooting

Ax machine maintenance
(including CO_2 absorbent)

Assist with Ax monitoring under
supervision of a technician

Sx room maintenance

Proper Sx pack maintenance
(clean, wrap, sterilize)

Front office skills

Proficient medical documentation

Prepare treatment plans (estimates)

Create an office visit
(DVM—not boarding/grooming)

Prepare Rx labels

Telephone skills

Greet clients

Technician level 1 skills mastery form

General nursing

Skill to be mastered	Completed	Date	Supervisor
Emergency response and preparedness			
Triage (telephone and clinical)			
Hospitalized patient care			
IVC maintenance			
U. catheter maintenance			
Fluid calculations			
Fluid additives			
Fluid selection knowledge			
Hygiene care for the ill or injured pet			
Nutritional support			
O_2 administration			
Nebulization			
Advanced vital signs (lung sounds, heart sounds, etc.)			
Monitoring patient ins/outs			
Doppler blood pressure measurement			
STT			
Tonometry			
Fluoroscein staining			
Cephalic blood collection			
Saphenous blood collection			
Jugular blood collection			
Endoscope cleaning and care			
Common disease knowledge			
Client communication (normal lab results, handle medical questions)			

Laboratory skills

Identify bacteria and yeast under microscope

Properly inoculate microbiology media

Identify contents in urine sediment

Prepare out-of-state laboratory specimens

Perform manual platelet count

Perform WBC differential

Identify RBC morphology

Perform bile acids testing

Collect specimen for c/s

Collect specimen for cytology

Understand CBC components

Understand chemistry test results

Anesthesia skills

Ax/pre-Ax calculations

Thorough understanding
of multiparameter monitoring

Use of suction

Dental scale and polish

Dental radiography

Assist routine surgeries

Identify, understand, and troubleshoot
monitor abnormalities

Ax vital sign documentation

Endotracheal tube extubation

Postoperative recovery

Technician level 2 skills mastery form

General nursing

Skill to be mastered	Completed	Date	Supervisor
Place IVC			
Place male u. cath			
Place female u. cath			
Place central venous catheter (femoral, saphenous)			
Calculate nutritional requirements			
Scrub into surgical procedures			
Cystocentesis via u/s			
FNA			
Extensive pathophysiology knowledge			
Diagnostic ECG			
Advanced endoscopy knowledge			
Care for PEG/EG tubes			
Care for thoracostomy tube			
Transfusion medicine			

Laboratory skills

ACTH stimulation test

Low-dose dex suppression testing

Prepare out-of-state laboratory specimens

Perform FNA

Blood culture collection and preparation

RBC fragility test

Saline agglutination test

Blood cross-matching

Anesthesia skills

Ax induction (under DVM supervision)

Endotracheal intubation

High-risk Ax patients, thoracic surgeries

Perform dental Ax blocks

Technician level 3 skills mastery form

General nursing

Skill to be mastered	Completed	Date	Supervisor
Properly place jugular central venous catheter			
Place IO catheter			
Arterial blood sample collection			
Arterial catheter placement			
Perform gastric lavage			
Perform gastrocentesis (GDV)			
Abdominocentesis			
Thoracocentesis			
Perform cystogram (cath, contrast media, etc.)			
Post-CPCR care/ICU nursing			
NG tube placement			
Nasal O_2 tube placement			
Peritoneal lavage			
Tracheotomy tube care			
Advanced transfusion medicine			
CRI calculations			

Laboratory skills

- Identify abnormal blood cells
- Identify abnormal FNA cells
- Evaluate CSF fluid
- Evaluate microbiology specimens
- Assist with bone marrow biopsy

Ten qualities of highly effective veterinary staff

Adapted from the Veterinary Healthcare Team of Arizona

Accountability

I am answerable for my actions.

Knowledge

I am eager to learn and understand.

Empathy

I am able to identify with the feelings of others.

Dedication

I am devoted to my purpose.

Professionalism

I conduct myself with confidence and competence.

Loyalty

I am faithful to the performance of my duties.

Respect

I am considerate of other people and things.

Responsibility

I have an ability to exercise control.

Positive Attitude

I am capable of maintaining a favorable mindset.

Tolerance

I allow others to express their differences.

Index

Note: Page entries followed by a "t" denote tables.

Clinical Small Animal Care: Promoting Patient Health through Preventative Nursing, First Edition.
Kimm Wuestenberg.
© 2012 John Wiley & Sons, Inc. Published 2012 by John Wiley & Sons, Inc.